Preventive Medicine in the United States
1900-1975

GEORGE ROSEN

PREVENTIVE MEDICINE
IN THE
UNITED STATES
1900-1975

TRENDS AND INTERPRETATIONS

1975   SCIENCE HISTORY PUBLICATIONS   NEW YORK

First published in the United States by
SCIENCE HISTORY PUBLICATIONS
a division of
Neale Watson Academic Publications, Inc.
156 Fifth Avenue, New York 10010

© SCIENCE HISTORY PUBLICATIONS 1975
First Edition 1975
(CIP Data on final page)
Designed and manufactured
in the U.S.A.

Contents

Preface

In July 1974, the Fogarty International Center, National Institutes of Health, invited the American College of Preventive Medicine to participate in the planning of a National Conference on Preventive Medicine which was held at the Center June 9-11, 1975. The objectives of the Conference were to examine preventive strategies and tactics applied to health problems in the United States in the recent past which had produced significant achievements, and to elicit from experts proposals for preventive measures which could lead to significant improvements in the health of the American people in the future.

Eight task forces working over a period of nine months prepared reports for inclusion in the published proceedings of the National Conference on Preventive Medicine. Subjects of these task force reports in addition to the present monograph on Preventive Medicine in the United States in Historical Perspective, included Prevention in Environmental Health, Prevention in Personal Health Services, Social Determinants of Human Health, Education and Training of Health Manpower for Prevention, Consumer Health Education, Quality Control and Evaluation, and Economic Impact of Preventive Medicine.

The monograph presented here was prepared as a background document for the Conference and is not intended to be a full-scale history. In line with the objective of tracing major trends in preventive medicine in the United States during the present century and interpreting the significance of current developments for future preventive action, only selected examples have been chosen for discussion and illustration. In terms of this objective a number of questions have been raised: Why have some forms of preventive action been effective while others have not? Why preventive measures have had to be applied indirectly in some instances? Why the existence of valid knowledge of disease etiology does not necessarily lead to effective prevention? How do social, economic, political and ideological elements facilitate or hinder preventive action? These and other issues provide the reason for this monograph, and the material presented in it provides some of the answers or at least indicates where they may be sought. For the reader who wishes to pursue the subject further there are over two hundred references to various aspects of preventive medicine.

I wish to thank Dr. Thomas D. Dublin (HRA) and Dr. Fred R. Mc-Crumb, Jr. (NIH) for their helpful comments and suggestions while this monograph was being prepared. I also want to express my appreciation particularly to Drs. William R. Barclay, C. Berry, Harold V. Ellingson, John W. Knutson and Carolyn A. Williams for their careful review of the initial draft of this monograph. Finally, I am grateful to the Fogarty International Center for permission to publish this monograph.

George Rosen, M.D., Ph. D.

Professor of the History of Medicine,
and Epidemiology and Public Health,
Yale University School of Medicine

Introduction

Action to prevent ill health and its consequences has been taken in one form or another from the earliest cultures up to the present. The operational expressions of such action have varied greatly, depending on the nature, organization and circumstances of the particular social group, and on the values, knowledge and technical means available to it.

Understanding the nature of a disease and of the causal elements involved in its occurrence can to a greater or lesser degree provide a basis for its prevention. Yet, more often than not, the application of such knowledge depends not only on the urgency and dimension of the health problem, but is frequently influenced to a significant extent by political, economic, cultural and ideological factors. Current instances are obvious in efforts to improve the nutrition of various groups of our population, to abate pollution of air and water, to protect workers in a wide range of occupations, as well as in the occurrence of outbreaks of diphtheria and poliomyelitis despite the availability of preventive means. Clearly, the existence of health problems does not automatically guarantee that action will be taken to prevent them, nor does availability of knowledge and technology always assure adequate application for prevention.

Despite such limitations, however, the desire to maintain health and prevent disease has led to activities at various levels of social organization as these seemed necessary, appropriate and effective for the desired end. This is the historical core of preventive medicine, involving as it does governmental policies and programs, private group undertakings, as well as family and individual actions with respect to health. An investigation of the evolution of preventive medicine in the United States from the turn of the century to the present can uncover forces and trends which have determined this process, and can thus provide a better understanding of our current situation as well as of possibilities for preventive action in the interest of health protection and promotion during the last quarter of the 20th century.

The Situation c. 1900

From the last decades of the 19th century to the present, a striking increase in the expectation of life occurred in the United States. The experience of Chicago between 1880 and 1950 aptly illustrates this trend.[1] During these seventy years, there was a dramatic decline in mortality rates. The consequence, based on a life-table analysis, was a gain in average length of life at birth of about 27 years for males and about 30 years for females. The increase was not as striking at all age levels, but was still of considerable magnitude even when the effect of infant mortality is omitted. During the period under consideration, the gain in life expectancy at one year of age was about 19 years for male children and around 24 years for female children.

This trend may be seen even more sharply in terms of survivor rates among a group of 10,000 persons. Of 10,000 male infants born in 1880, 8,037 survived the first year of life; in 1950 almost the same number, 8,003, attained the age of 55. In 1880, 5,844 males (58%) reached age 25, while in 1950, 5,790 (58%) survived to age 65. This shift is even more marked among females. In 1880, 8,489 female infants attained one year of age. A slightly larger number (8,736) survived to age 55 in 1950. Furthermore, the number of women who reached the age of 65 in 1950 was more than twice that in 1880.

With variations, the experience of Chicago has been that of other American communities during this period, and indeed of the country as a whole. At the turn of the century, the average expectation of life at birth was 49.2 years; by 1966, it was 70.1. In 1900, at age 5, the average child could expect to live an additional 55 years; by 1966, a 5-year old could expect an additional 67.1 years, or a gain of 12.1 years.

The increase in life expectancy at birth can be traced mainly to a decline in infant and child mortality, that is, between birth and age 15. Only a smaller proportion of the gain in years can be attributed to a reduction in mortality among those over the age of 25. This is clearly evident from the following table.[2]

Average Number of Years of Life Remaining at Specified Ages:
United States, 1900-02 and 1966

AGE AT BEGINNING OF YEAR	Average number of years of life remaining		Increase in average remaining lifetime (in years)
	1900-02	1966	
Birth	49.2	70.1	20.9
1	55.2	70.8	15.6
5	55.0	67.1	12.1
25	39.1	48.0	8.9
65	11.9	14.6	2.7

3

An understanding of the profound changes in the mortality picture during the past 70 years must take account of the causes of sickness and death throughout this period, of their changing incidence and prevalence, and of the reasons for these developments. At the beginning of the 20th century, the most pressing health problems centered on the high morbidity and mortality due to communicable diseases. In 1900, the leading causes of death were influenza and pneumonia, tuberculosis, and infections of the gastrointestinal tract, together accounting for almost one-third of all deaths. Typhoid fever outbreaks were still common, although its importance as a cause of death had declined since the middle of the 19th century. Malaria still occurred in northern states such as New York and New Jersey, but was most widely prevalent in the southern United States. Diphtheria ranked tenth among the causes of death, but it was a major source of mortality among children, while other transmissible diseases such as measles, whooping cough, scarlet fever, rheumatic fever, meningococcal infections and syphilis added to the burden of illness and death in this age group.[3]

Although mortality from communicable diseases was high at the turn of the century, nevertheless the situation had improved since the latter 19th century. A comparison of the prevalence of some infectious diseases in the middle of the 19th century and the early decades of the present century reveals a remarkable contrast. In the 19th century, epidemic outbreaks of certain diseases such as diarrhea and dysentery, typhoid fever, smallpox, diphtheria, scarlet fever as well as others, occurred regularly and tended to keep the gross mortality high.[4] The wide variation in the annual death rates, a marked characteristic of this period, was due to these outbreaks. In Chicago, for example, during the decade 1850-1859, the mortality rate for scarlet fever varied from a maximum of 272 per 100,000 to a minimum of six. As mortality rates declined, they also became steadier. The magnitude of this decline may be seen from a comparison of the maximal rates since 1850 with those in the 1920s for some of the diseases mentioned above.

CHICAGO	Death rate per 100,000 population	
Diseases	Highest rate since 1850	Highest rate in the 1920s
Diarrhea and Dysentery	603	81
Diphtheria	291	24
Scarlet Fever	272	7
Smallpox	230	0.5
Typhoid fever	174	2
Malaria	106	0.2
Whooping Cough	92	6
Measles	80	7

4

Alongside the communicable diseases, there were also other morbid conditions of considerable importance as causes of illness and death in specific population groups. Grover F. Powers, the Yale pediatrician, observed in 1939 that until about 1925 "the majority of admissions to any non-contagious children's ward were due either to diarrhea or to the results of vitamin D deficiency."[5]

Non-infectious diarrhea of infants and very young children was perhaps the most dreaded and prevalent of the diseases affecting the urban child. Poverty and parental ignorance in conjunction with a lack of knowledge among physicians of the normal and pathological physiology of infancy produced a veritable slaughter of babies each summer. This situation did not improve materially until the later 1920s after clinical and laboratory studies demonstrated that the infants were suffering from fluid loss, electrolyte imbalance and circulatory failure, knowledge which was applied for prevention and therapy. Thus, in Connecticut, the deathrate under one year from diarrhea per 1000 live births dropped from 23.1 in 1916 to 8.6 in 1923, to 1.9 in 1936. Similar experiences occurred in other American states and cities.[6]

During the later 19th and early 20th centuries, rickets, the other disease mentioned by Powers, was widespread in urban communities, especially in slum districts, though the children of the more affluent were not exempt. William Osler noted in 1901 that in Vienna and London from 50 to 80 percent of all children seen in clinics had signs of rickets. He also observed that the disease was highly prevalent in American cities, particularly among the children of black and Italian families.[7] Twenty years later, in 1921, E.V. McCollum claimed that probably one half of the children in the cities of the United States either had or had had rickets.[8] The disease was rarely fatal in itself, but rachitic children readily died of pneumonia secondary to thoracic deformities, and less often of convulsions due to rachitic tetany or spasm of the larynx. Deformity of the pelvis in female children often led to difficulties in parturition when they reached adulthood, thus adding to illness and death during the childbearing years.

But there were no clear ideas on the etiology of the disease during the early years of the present century. Osler, for example, refers to lack of sunlight and fresh air as predisposing causes, and hardly mentions preventive measures, except by implication. He suggests cod-liver oil only half-heartedly, among a number of other therapeutic recommendations. In 1918, Noël Paton and Leonard Findlay summed up the state of knowledge on the etiology of rickets with the statement: "The cause of rickets is still undetermined," a position underscored in 1919 by Sir George Newman in his statement on the role of preventive medicine in a national health policy.[9] During this very period, however, between 1918 and 1924, the demonstration of a heat stable, antirachitic factor by E.V. McCollum in America and Edward Mellanby in

England made it possible to solve the riddle and to mount a campaign for its prevention (see below).[10]

Rickets was not the only health problem affecting preschool and school children. In fact, it was but one major consequence of the large, widespread problem of malnutrition among children and its deleterious effects on their physical and intellectual development. Robert Hunter, in his study of poverty in 1904, estimated that in New York alone some sixty or seventy thousand children went hungry to school, leading in many instances to poor class-work.[11] This and other findings were reinforced by John Spargo in his book *The Bitter Cry of the Children* (1906). He found that sanitary regulations had produced some improvement of child health, but also that thousands of slum children were undernourished and racked by tuberculosis, rickets and other diseases.[12]

Awareness of dental disease as a health problem of children and adults was already present early in the century. In 1900, the National Dental Association (in 1922 it became the American Dental Association) established a Committee on Oral Hygiene in Our Public Schools for the purpose of teaching "Good Teeth, Good Health" to school children. The Committee urged state dental societies to organize oral hygiene committees to compile statistics on the prevalence of dental caries among children and to teach them oral hygiene. This concern with prophylaxis was further fueled by belief in a relationship between dental pathology and other diseases. As expressed by William Hunter in 1909, "The worst cases of anemia, gastritis, of obscure fevers of unknown origin, of numerous disturbances of all kinds, ranging from mental depression up to actual lesions of the cord, of chronic rheumatic affections, of kidney disease, are those which owe their origin to, or are gravely complicated by, the oral sepsis."[13]

Reports during the same period provided evidence that the prevalence of dental disease was a consequence not just of malnutrition but of a wider complex of problems produced by poverty. Of 391 workingmen's families in New York City studied by Robert C. Chapin in 1907, only 16 percent reported expenditures for dental work. The study revealed "a deplorable lack of attention to the teeth on the part of the large majority in all income groups," but also showed that "the percentage of families that do pay the dentist increases, however, with increase of income."[14] Among 2,598 families surveyed by the Health Insurance Commission of Illinois in 1918-1919, only 981, about 38 percent, reported having had any dental service during the year.[15]

Illness and death among pregnant and parturient women also began to attract attention during this period, although the precise dimensions of the problem were not quite clear owing to unsatisfactory statistical data. For all practical purposes prenatal care did not exist in the first decade of the century. The supervision of pregnancy even among the private patients of leading

6

obstetricians was generally only meager and casual. Hardly any effort was made to foresee and prevent complications that might affect either mother or child.[16] Nor was the situation much better in hospitals. As one medical observer noted in 1909:

> "Of the maternity hospitals, it is still unhappily true that they are regarded largely as clinics for the edification of young physicians. With two or three splendid exceptions, the maternity hospitals of New York have no adequate provision for the protection of mothers before childbirth or for following them to their homes after they have been discharged."[17]

Many women delivered their babies without any medical attendance.[18] Midwives were employed extensively, especially among mothers of foreign birth and in isolated rural communities, and many were ignorant or poorly trained. A study by Anna E. Rude, of the Children's Bureau, revealed in 1923 that in 31 states there were 26, 627 midwives officially allowed to practice, but that more than 17,000 unauthorized midwives were practicing in these and other states.[19] Small wonder that in 1917 out of 16 "progressive" nations, the United States ranked fourteenth in the maternal death rate.[20] Awareness of a need to deal with maternal morbidity and mortality was reinforced by recognizing that infancy could not be protected without the protection of maternity, one of the principles on which the Children's Bureau developed its program, following its establishment in 1912.[21] What this meant concretely is clear from the report of S. Josephine Baker in 1913 that in New York City 35 percent of the infant mortality was related to the health status of the mother during pregnancy and parturition.[22] Interest in the prevention of maternal deaths increased during the second decade of the century, due in no small measure to the educational efforts of the Children's Bureau and its investigations of the causes, which began to provide a firm basis for action. Puerperal septicemia, the largest single cause of maternal mortality, in 1920 responsible for about 34 percent of all such deaths, was considered particularly suitable for preventive action. The desire to reduce and if possible to eliminate such preventable causes of maternal morbidity and mortality was in part responsible for the enactment in 1921 of the Maternity and Infancy (Sheppard-Towner) Act, which was to provide an important base for prevention.

Effective concern with occupational health is of relatively recent origin in the United States.[23] In 1900, the field of occupational health was still *terra incognita* to most Americans including the medical profession. When Alice Hamilton attended the Fourth International Congress on Occupational Accidents and Diseases at Brussels in 1910, she heard Dr. Gilbert of the Belgian Labor Department dispose of the Americans with the curt statement, "It is well known that there is no industrial hygiene in the United States, Ca n'existe pas."[24] The accuracy of this judgment was confirmed the same year by Henry W. Farnam in opening the First National Conference on Industrial Diseases in Chicago. "Our country is just beginning to appreciate the importance of industrial hygiene," he said, and went on to describe the situation of those concerned with the health of workers as being "like that of a watchman on a high tower. He does not know exactly how the attack is to be made but he knows enough to justify him in giving the alarm and in advising that scouts be sent out to ascertain more precisely the strength and position of the foe."[25] However, the decade 1910 to 1920 saw the establishment of occupational health as a significant field of action in terms of research and the application of the results to prevention. Emerging developments during this period were the product of a cumulative movement extending back over several decades and influenced in some degree by European experience.

The roots of this movement can be traced to the latter decades of the 19th century and were nourished in a broad sense by the quest for social justice that characterized the first decades of the present century. One of these roots was the governmental machinery that had been created after the Civil War, first by the states and then by the federal government to deal with the interests and problems of the wage earner. The state labor bureaus were agencies for investigating labor conditions and making recommendations to legislatures. The worker's health was one of the problems that early attracted the attention of these bureaus. The effect of occupation upon health was touched on in studies published by New Jersey (1883), Wisconsin (1887-1888), and Montana (1893). Between 1889 and 1895, New Jersey published a series of reports dealing with the effect of occupation upon longevity.[26] These studies continued into the 20th century as evidenced, for example, by W.C. Garrison's report in 1905 on health conditions in the pottery industry in Trenton, New Jersey, one of a series on diseases and disease tendencies in industries of that state.[27] These agencies also provided a useful basis for an attack on the conditions under which women and children were employed, and on the health consequences which they entailed. Thus, in 1909, a U.S. Senate *Report on Condition of Women and Child Wage Earners in the United States* emphasized the conditions in the glass, textile, clothing and other industries which produced illnesses among women and children as a result of poor ventilation, noise, speed, excessively long hours and related conditions.

A number of events, all occurring in 1910 provide further evidence of growing attention to occupational health. That eventful year saw not only the convening of the first National Conference on Industrial Diseases, but also the creation of the United States Bureau of Mines, the establishment by W. Gilman Thompson of the first clinic for occupational diseases at the Cornell Medical College in New York, the publication by John B. Andrews of his studies on phosphorus poisoning in the American match industry, the appearance of Alice Hamilton's report on industrial lead poisoning, and the issuance by the United States Bureau of Labor of a list of industrial poisons. The same year the joint Board of Sanitary Control of the Cloak, Suit and Skirt Industry of Greater New York began the study and control of health conditions in clothing factories and shops. The U.S. Public Health Service also began in 1910 to take cognizance of dangers to health in the working environment and of the need to prevent them, so that four years later a Division of Industrial Hygiene and Sanitation, headed by J.W. Schereschewsky was set up. That year, 1914, Schereschewsky studied the health of garment workers in New York City, revealing an excessive prevalence of tuberculosis.[28] Finally, mention must be made of the pioneer work of George M. Kober, who in 1908 prepared the first American text on industrial health.[29]

Clearly, by 1910, a number of socially conscious Americans—economists, physicians, labor leaders, lawyers, social scientists and others—were aware that problems of occupational disease were not receiving adequate attention, and efforts had been started to improve the situation. By the second decade of the 20th century, the movement to better health conditions in industry was in full swing.[30]

Accidents and injuries, particularly on the job, represented a significant part of the burden of death, illness and disability borne by the American people in 1900. The total number of deaths from accidents and injuries reported during the census year 1900 was 57,513, which ranked seventh among the ten leading causes of death, an indication of the seriousness of the problem. Yet these figures do not reveal its actual dimensions which were much greater, since they omit those who were injured and recovered, in numerous cases with permanent impairments. In 1900, for example, deaths from railway accidents numbered 7,865, but there were also 50,320 persons injured, a total of 58,185. In 1906, the total was 108,324 (10,618 killed; 97,706 injured).[31] Even more revealing are figures collected by Frederick L. Hoffman, statistician for the Prudential Life Insurance Company. During the year 1913, there were approximately 25,000 fatal accidents, 300,000 serious injuries, and 2,000,000 other injuries among workers in the United States. Furthermore, according to Gordon L. Berry of the National Committee for the Prevention of Blindness, in 1917 of the 2,000,000 annual non-fatal accidents, about 200,000 involved the eyes, and approximately 15,000 persons were blinded as a result of industrial accidents.[32]

The health problems of industrial workers and their accident experience, as well as that of other groups in the population, reflect the revolution in the technology of production, communication and transportation, as well as in business and industrial organization, which followed the Civil War and has continued through the 20th century. Illustrative is the case of the automobile. In 1900, there were an estimated 8,000 "horseless carriages" in the United States. By 1921, 9,346,195 motor vehicles were registered, and by 1925 the number had increased to 17,496,420.[33] The introduction of the automobile created a new environment with new hazards, and as the number

9

of automobiles increased, so did the deaths and injuries. Even though the statistical data for the period from 1900 to the mid-1920s are defective, the general trend is clear. The death rate per 100,000 from automobile accidents rose from 1.0 in 1900-1910, to 17.9 in 1926, increasing approximately eighteen times.[34] Motor vehicle deaths increased from 2.2 percent of all accidental deaths in 1910 to 20.5 percent in 1924. By the mid-1920s the existence of a new health problem was evident. As R.S. Stoeckel, Commissioner of Motor Vehicles in Connecticut, said in 1926,

> "The traffic accident is part of the public health problem. . . . As compared with smallpox, diphtheria, typhoid or with any other epidemic disease and as compared with accidental injury and death from any other cause, it runs close to the top, with every prospect of heading the list within another year. So its place and right to consideration in every public health movement in the future is assured and those health agencies and organizations which have as their special duty the general supervision of the public health will all take active interest in it."[35]

Concern with the relation of environmental conditions to ill health was not limited to industrial workers. It was recognized that the health of the worker in the plant could not be compartmentalized. Conditions of life in the home as well as conditions in the factory could deleteriously affect the worker's health so that effective prevention required action along several interrelated lines. As a basic element of the standard of living which affected not only the worker but also the household, housing was particularly important and was intimately linked with poverty and disease, especially in slum districts and among the urban poor. The nature of the slum economy and the role of housing in it had already been recognized by the mid-19th century, and efforts to improve housing as a means of preventing disease had been undertaken before 1900.[36] Despite some improvement after 1865, the housing situation around the turn of the century was still deplorable for the working poor and immigrants. The urgent need for housing reform, especially in connection with tenements, was emphasized preeminently in terms of the prevalence of tuberculosis, even though the occurrence of other diseases such as typhoid fever and diphtheria was also mentioned frequently. As John H. Pryor, the Health Commissioner of Buffalo, expressed this view, "Now tuberculosis reigns, and the record of suffering and death is almost unparalleled;" the disease must be attacked by depriving it of its "natural breeding place," the dark crowded tenement.[37] This required improved, sanitary housing, a view shared by many others.[38]

Not only was the emphasis in 1900 on the relation between tenements and tuberculosis a recognition of an important social and health problem, it was also most appropriate in a wider symbolic sense. Tuberculosis was the epitome of urban maladies, the mirror of a community's mode of life and the milieu in which that life was passed, revealing the deprivation, dirt and disease which pervaded the existence of so many people. Robert Koch's discovery in 1882 of the tubercle bacillus as the specific etiologic agent in tuberculosis did not immediately lead to its prevention and control. What it did was provide a means of opening up the complex of interdependent causative factors, and make possible an understanding of the ways in which social conditions and biological factors interacted to produce the disease, and of the means necessary to deal with them.[39] Regarded as social allies of the tubercle bacillus, fostering the occurrence and propagation of the disease, were poverty and low living standards, poor housing and overcrowded dwellings, unsanitary working conditions, ignorance and poor hygienic practices.

Three intertwining developments in American society during the last decades of the 19th century and the early decades of the 20th century produced the economic and social world in which these factors operated. Industrial expansion, urban growth, and a flood of immigration all combined to produce conditions where thousands of people huddled in unbelievably inadequate housing deprived of some of the most elementary requirements of civilized life.

From 1860 to 1910 the urban portion of the population rose from 19 to 45 percent of the total, due in large measure to the immigrants who poured into the cities and industrial towns where workers were in demand.[40] The immigrants had left the backward, wretched circumstances of countryside and hamlet in southern and eastern Europe, from which the majority came, to seek a better life in the New World. Most, however, were unskilled and had to accept poorly paid jobs performing heavy manual labor. But even the skilled worked excessively long hours for low wages under unhealthful conditions. Frequently, they worked for their compatriots, often as subcontractors, converting their dwellings into sweatshops employing all the members of a family.

Immigration from Europe tended to overshadow another significant population shift in the United States which began during this period and was to have major repercussions just before, during and after the Second World War. From the turn of the century into the 1900s, economic distress, disfranchisement and dissatisfaction with the pattern of race relations and violence to which they were subjected drove thousands of blacks to move north. As early as 1903, W.E.B. Du Bois noted that "the most significant economic change among Negroes in the last ten or twenty years had been their influx into northern cities." According to the census of 1910, two cities, New York and Washington, had over 90,000 Negroes, and three others, Philadelphia, Baltimore and New Orleans, over 80,000. This trend was reinforced by the First World War, when Southern Negroes went North in large numbers to look for jobs in the booming war industries. During the years 1916-1918, an estimated 400,000 blacks suddenly moved North.[41] The North, however, was no land of milk and honey, and the experience of the black migrants was similar to that of the European immigrants but with even more severe discrimination.

Thus, around the turn of the century, the growing cities of the United States were increasingly confronted by problems most often associated with the movement of population. The inescapable reality of these problems, plus a growing conviction of the need for social change to avoid violent disruption of the existing order, led to a broad movement of reform dedicated to the eradication of demonstrable social ills and the realization through planned social action of conditions for a better life. From this standpoint campaigns were mounted to deal with a wide range of problems: poverty and dependency, tenement house reform, sweatshops, child labor, juvenile delinquency, prostitution and others, among which ill health was prominent as a cause or a consequence.[42]

The great importance of health problems within this complex context was well recognized. In 1909, Edward T. Devine, secretary of the New York Charity Organization Society, not only noted that "Ill health is perhaps the most constant of the attendants of poverty," but went on to emphasize that

"An inquiry into the physical condition of the members of the families that ask for aid . . . clearly indicates that whether it be the first cause or merely a complication from the effect of other causes, physical disability is at any rate a very serious disabling condition at the time of application in three-fourths . . . of all the families that come under the care of the Charity Organization Society, who are probably in no degree exceptional among families in need of charitable aid."[43]

An aversion to human suffering and a desire to prevent, abate or ameliorate the circumstances which produced misery for so many were not new around 1900. These attitudes, along with other factors, had been integral elements in the movements for sanitary and factory reform in the 19th century. According to the tenets of economic liberalism, however, it was believed during most of the nineteenth century that increased production resulting from industrial advance would banish scarcity, and as a result eliminate poverty and decrease misery as far as possible. Yet, the inescapable fact, at the turn of the century, of poverty, disease, vice and their consequences as large scale urban phenomena, and an increasing awareness that these seemingly were symptoms of a more deep-seated social malaise, made it increasingly impossible to rest content with the earlier belief. From the discontents and disorders that plagued not only the United States but other industrial nations as well, there developed a stream of dissenting opinion manifesting itself concretely in various proposals and programs for reform. In all of these there was a shift away from the freely competitive order to an acceptance, to a greater or lesser degree, of the necessity for state interference. Government intervention in the interests of community health and welfare had been developing throughout the 19th century, but it was only toward the end of this period and the early years of this century that this trend was formulated as a theory and program of social action.

The state was conceived by reformers to be an indispensable instrument for achieving desirable social goals. At the same time, this philosophy did not exclude voluntary action by independent citizens. Indeed, in many instances public action in the form of legislation and regulation was obtained only after agitation by voluntary organizations. The ideological thrust of this movement was characteristically expressed by Walter Lippmann in 1914:

"We can no longer treat life," he wrote, "as something that has trickled down to us. We have to deal with it deliberately, devise its social organization, alter its tools, formulate its method, educate and control it. In endless ways, we put intention where custom has reigned. We break up routines, make decisions, choose our ends, select means."[44]

The orientation of the reform movement in the United States was pragmatic and empirical, deeply imbued with confidence in what might be accomplished by rational social action. There was no rigid system of ideas that had to be accepted in its entirety by those who participated, a view clearly expressed by Edward T. Devine when he observed that the movement was

"neither reactionary nor Utopian. Both liberal progressives and social-minded conservatives had part in it. Its embryonic philosophy was so formulated as not to exclude any who were willing to face the facts and to cooperate for the eradication of demonstrable evils, for the realization of demonstrable possibilities for a happier and better life, for the essentials of rational human existence for all."[45]

Conservation, Efficiency, Prevention
And Social Action:
Ideologies and Concepts

The reasons for this orientation are not hard to find. The desire to create a social environment in which individuals could achieve maximum physical, mental and cultural development grew out of an increasing awareness that the United States had become an industrial society in which deepening cleavages were developing between the upper and lower classes and preventing the fulfillment of the American promise for the latter, many of whom had emigrated to the United States to improve their lot. To prevent further exacerbation of this situation, and as far as possible to close the rents in the social fabric, it was necessary to establish national responsibility for health and welfare. As Herbert Croly wrote in 1909, "to unite the Hamiltonian principle of national political responsibility and efficiency with a frank democratic purpose" would give a new power to democracy.[46]

Since poverty and its associated ills were caused by social maladjustments, governmental action was required to alter the circumstances and to eliminate the factors creating the problems. This meant setting standards for income, working conditions, housing, quality of food, and health care.[47] Mary K. Simkhovitch in 1917 insisted on the need to "recognize and establish standards of health, education, leisure and income" and emphasized that an income standard was a "social necessity in just the sense and for precisely the same reason as is a cubic air space standard."[48] The endeavor to set criteria for a normal standard of living coincided at several points with the conservation movement of the period in its aim to prevent disease and death and to promote national health.

Toward the end of the 19th century, social critics began to campaign vigorously against the private exploitation of the national wealth and for protection of the environment. Conservation became a popular crusading idea and an important American ideology early in this century, and in June 1908 President Theodore Roosevelt appointed a Federal Commission on the Conservation of Natural Resources.[49] For conservationists who advocated planned use and scientific management of natural resources and national wealth, it was clear that health was a resource not to be overlooked. The crusade for the conservation of human resources was initiated by two economists, J. Pease Norton and Irving Fisher, both of Yale University. In 1906, at a meeting of the American Association for the Advancement of Science, Norton read a paper advocating a national department of health. In support of this proposal, he stressed the losses to society arising from preventable illness which could be reduced by such an agency.[50] In consequence, the AAAS set up a Committee of One Hundred on National Health with Fisher as president and Norton as executive secretary, and the drive for national action was under way.[51] The Committee conducted inquiries and endeavored to secure support from leading politicians, public officials, representatives of public health, medicine and social welfare as well as business, labor and agriculture. Information collected from a wide range of sources was presented to the National Conservation Commission as reports concerning problems related to the preservation of health.[52] Most important was *A Report on National Vitality Its Wastes and Conservation* prepared by Fisher in 1908 and submitted to the Conservation Commission of which he was also a member. Fisher urged the federal and state governments, as well as the municipalities, to undertake vigorous action to protect the people from disease, and thus conserve a basic national resource. "It is both bad policy and bad economy to leave this work mainly to the weak and spasmodic efforts of charity, or to the philanthropy of physicians". Furthermore, the federal government should "provide more and greater laboratories for research in preventive medicine and public hygiene. Provision should also be made for better and more universal vital statistics, without which it is impossible to know the exact conditions in an epidemic, or, in general, the sanitary or insanitary conditions in any part of the country." Fisher was a strong advocate of measures to protect the health of mothers and children, and stressed the need for school health programs. He urged the importance of dealing with environmental pollution (smoke, dust, noxious gases, noise), as well as with such social evils as alcoholism and prostitution.[53] Fisher's *Report* is clearly a product of his time in terms of knowledge, but the principles which he advocated adumbrate the shape of numerous developments in succeeding decades. He recognized the complex interdependence of industrial society, and held that social interest superseded individual interests in such matters as resource conservation, health promotion, disease prevention, sanitation and the like. The circumstance that social and health problems in the United States were not simply local matters meant that action was needed within the broad framework of a national policy. Fisher viewed such a policy as the product of humanitarianism linked with national interest.

Certainly, it is no accident that such views achieved prominence in a period marked by a resurgence of mercantilist ideas and policies in the United States, by efforts to acquire colonies, to secure markets and sources of raw materials, and to have a large productive population. If an industrial power wanted a productive labor force, if it wanted enough healthy fit men to serve in its armed forces, conservation of its human resources was necessary. This view was reinforced in the United States during the First World War when the consequences of neglecting the national health became evident in the large number of rejected draftees, an experience England had already endured at the time of the Boer War. Many young men examined for military service were found to be physically unfit, a situation that recurred in the Second World War.[54]

The connection between national interest, resource conservation, and health protection was clearly and succinctly put by the National Conservation Commission in the statement that "Natural resources are of no avail without men and women to develop them, and only a strong and sound citizenship can make a nation permanently great. We cannot too soon enter on the duty of conserving our chief source of strength by the prevention of disease and the prolongation of life".[55] A similar attitude is expressed by the motto of the American Association for Labor Legislation: "The fundamental purpose of labor legislation is the conservation of the human resources of the nation."

Central to any program of action was the idea that prevention was feasible. According to Pease Norton in 1906, there were four great wastes, "preventable death, preventable sickness, preventable conditions of low physical and mental efficiency, and preventable ignorance," and all of these were unnecessary.[56] The keynote for the period was struck by Hermann Biggs in 1911. "Disease is largely a removable evil," he wrote.

"It continues to afflict humanity, not only because of incomplete knowledge of its causes and lack of individual and public hygiene, but also because it is extensively fostered by harsh economic and industrial conditions and by wretched housing in congested communities. These conditions and consequently the diseases which spring from them can be removed by better social organization. No duty of society, acting through its governmental agencies, is paramount to this obligation to attack the removable causes of disease."[57]

The notion that disease could be prevented by appropriate action was certainly not new in the 20th century. The idea had been accepted from the earliest times, and various means had been employed to make it a reality. Until the later 19th century, however, such actions were based overwhelmingly on tradition, empiricism and faith. Even measures recognized as effective, such as vaccination against smallpox and the use of citrus fruits to prevent scurvy, had no scientific basis to explain their effectiveness or to indicate whether such principles could be used for other diseases. When Lemuel Shattuck wrote in 1850 that "If consumption is ever to be eradicated it can only be done by preventive means and not by cure," he was expressing his faith in a possibility and presenting a challenge to the future for its realization. Not quite 50 years later, however, the view that diseases could be prevented was being spread to the medical profession and the lay public, and was being acted upon with a characteristic optimism that means were now available to effectively prevent or control the hazards and ravages of infections and other diseases, an optimistic view resting on a more solid foundation than hope and faith. This trend is already evident at the end of the 19th century. On August 15, 1890, Henry B. Baker, a physician who was secretary of the Michigan State Board of Health, addressed the Sanitary

Convention of the state on the restriction and prevention of dangerous diseases. "The diseases which can be restricted," he said,

"are those which are *communicable*. The 'communicable' diseases include those which are contagious, those which are infectious, those which are in any way communicated or spread from one person to another, such diseases as smallpox, scarlet fever, diphtheria, measles and whooping cough. ...At least one of the most dangerous of all diseases, namely, consumption, has in recent years been found to be a communicable disease and a preventable disease. There is considerable evidence now tending to prove that pneumonia is a communicable disease, and that probably many deaths from that disease could be prevented by the general adoption of measures which recent investigations have revealed.... We thus gain some idea of the vast importance of this subject—the restriction and prevention of the dangerous communicable diseases.... Especially do we appreciate the importance of this subject when we consider that we absolutely know that a large proportion of the cases and deaths from the most of these diseases are *preventable*, and we believe that this is true of all of these diseases."[58]

That Baker's was not an isolated view is evident from a paper on the prevention of disease read by William W. Potter before the New York Academy of Medicine on February 1, 1894. Stressing the theme that prevention is the preeminent function of "the physician of modern times," he called attention to the problems requiring major attention. Noting that "some of the exanthematous fevers have not now the same dread to humanity as formerly, since the triumph in medicine in solving the methods of their prevention and cure," yet "there is being added to the list a number of maladies that formerly were not thought to be contagious, or at least infectious, but have now become well known to be so through the investigations and studies of clinicians and men experienced in the science of bacteriology."[59] Potter supported his contention by discussing four diseases: tuberculosis, typhoid fever, diphtheria, and gonorrheal infection in women. Much remained to be clarified in these conditions, yet enough information was available already for appropriate measures to be taken, recognizing of course that modifications might have to be made on the basis of new knowledge derived from research. But action was necessary because "consumption, diphtheria, typhoid fever, and gonorrhea are slaying or invaliding *unnecessarily* hundreds of thousands annually."[60]

Within the next two decades the advocacy of disease prevention became even more fervent, expressing an increasing recognition that effective weapons to combat preventable diseases were in hand. On December 10, 1910, Eugene H. Porter, Health Commissioner of New York State, addressed the Association of Life Insurance Presidents at their annual meeting in Chicago.

17

Porter's subject was the fight against preventable diseases, and his aim was to enlist the insurance companies in this effort. His basic premise was that "The last fifty years have seen more progress made in knowledge of the causes of diseases than all the centuries before," so that "now we have a new foundation and a new knowledge and we are living in the midst of a great remaking of medical history."[61] This assertion is borne out by Milton J. Rosenau in the preface to his classic text, *Preventive Medicine and Hygiene*, published in 1913. "The progress in hygiene and sanitation has been so rapid," he wrote, "that the subject of preventive medicine has become a specialty, and its scope has become so broad that the question throughout the making of this book has been rather, what to leave out than what to include."[62]

Within the concept of preventable diseases, Porter included not only the communicable diseases, but also cancer, accidents and homicide. Nor was he an exception. In 1909, Woods Hutchinson, clinical professor of medicine at the New York Polyclinic, published a volume on preventable diseases for the lay public, in which he devoted chapters to appendicitis, rheumatism, cancer and nervous conditions as well as to tuberculosis, typhoid fever and other communicable diseases.[63] Rosenau included heredity, eugenics and occupational diseases, as well as prevention of the communicable diseases.

Americans shared this broad concept of prevention with foreigners. On July 20, 1905, the Scottish psychiatrist, Sir James Crichton-Browne, addressed the Preventive Medicine Section of the London Congress of the Royal Institute of Health on the prevention of senility. "Glancing at the subjects of discussion arranged for this section," he commented,

"one would infer that preventive medicine is for the young... It is no doubt in early years that preventive medicine has achieved its greatest triumphs, can in several departments be carried out, and may confer protective influences that last far on in life; but there is, or ought to be, no limit to its operations, and as it is directed against not only disease and death, but degeneration and decay, it should continue its services as long as morbific agencies assail the organism."[64]

A similarly broad approach to prevention was taken by Sir George Newman in 1919 in his national program for preventive medicine. Under non-infectious conditions, he specifically included heart disease, rickets, mental disease, dental caries, indigestion and alimentary disease and preventive surgery. In addition he also discussed health and physical education as well as research in preventive medicine.[65]

But how were these ideas and concepts to be realized in practice? What knowledge was available during the early decades of this century that could be applied to disease prevention and health promotion? Who was to apply this knowledge, by what means, and under what circumstances? Which existing institutions could be used or did new ones have to be created? What was the responsibility of government at various levels, of citizen groups and of individuals in prevention of disease and the promotion of health? These and other related questions were tackled during the period from 1910 to 1940, and answers were developed that had definite consequences for the period following World War II.

Knowledge and Its Applications:
Institutions, Personnel and Techniques

By the last two decades of the 19th century, light was being cast on the etiology of the communicable diseases by demonstrating specific causative organisms in many instances. Within a few years, largely between 1876 and 1898, armed with methods devised chiefly by Robert Koch, the microbial causes of numerous human and animal diseases were revealed, among them typhoid, malaria, tuberculosis, diphtheria, dysentery, tetanus, and cholera. Until the 1880s, microbes had been shown to be the probable or certain etiological agents in only a few diseases. Obermeier (1867/68) had shown that a spiral organism was consistently present in cases of relapsing fever and that the disease was transmissible; Koch in 1876 had demonstrated the causal role of the anthrax bacillus; and in 1879 Neisser discovered the gonococcus. Then with the 1880s the golden age of bacteriological discovery was ushered in. As if a dam had burst, causative organisms of various diseases were demonstrated in rapid succession, often several in one year.[66]

Nonetheless, certain problems remained. In some diseases, such as typhoid fever and cholera, new cases did occur in persons who had had no direct contact with individuals affected by the disease. In other conditions, however, persons who had been exposed to contact with sick individuals remained unaffected. Light was finally thrown upon these obscurities during the closing decade of the 19th century and the first decade of the 20th by a number of brilliant investigations that revealed the part played by vectors, or intermediaries, in the transmission of communicable diseases. As early as 1855, Pettenkofer had suggested that healthy human carriers could transmit cholera, but it was not until the end of the century that this hypothesis was substantiated and the significance of the human carrier recognized. Between 1893 and 1900 this mode of transmission was demonstrated for cholera, diphtheria, and typhoid, and by 1910, when C.V. Chapin published his classic work on *The Sources and Modes of Infection*, the role of the human carrier was securely established. Paralleling these contributions was the equally important demonstration of the role of the animal vector. Following the work of Theobald Smith and F.L. Kilborne on Texas cattle fever demonstrating that ticks feeding on infected cattle transmitted the pathogenic protozoan, *Piroplasma bigeminum*, the animal carrier had to be considered in disease transmission. In subsequent years this method of transmission was demonstrated in other important communicable diseases, among them malaria, plague, yellow fever, dengue, Rocky Mountain spotted fever, epidemic typhus, murine typhus, Colorado Tick fever and rickettsial pox.

Concurrently, microbiology profoundly affected the concepts and practices of preventive medicine and public health as practised around the

20

turn of the century through the development and application of immunology. The artificial production of immunity had been known for more than 100 years, having been employed for the prevention of smallpox, first through the introduction of variolation and later by the discovery and application of Jennerian vaccination. The essential principle that a mild case of the disease protected the individual from further attacks, even when the infection is potent, was employed empirically without any understanding of the underlying mechanism. The development of protective vaccines by Louis Pasteur (chicken cholera, 1881; swine erysipelas, 1883; rabies, 1884/85) stimulated interest in the phenomenon of immunity, and led investigators to look for the mechanisms that inoculation set in motion. By the end of the 19th century it had become evident that a high degree of resistance to the causative organisms of certain communicable diseases could be produced by the injection of these germs in an attenuated live state or when dead, or by inoculation with extracts from such organisms. At the same time it was found that the blood of immunized animals and humans contained substances, antibodies, that had significant prophylactic and therapeutic powers when injected into healthy or sick persons. Pasteur's discovery of prophylactic vaccines was followed by the development of others for such diseases as plague, cholera, typhoid and paratyphoid, tuberculosis, yellow fever, pertussis, and more recently poliomyelitis and measles. Immune sera were also developed for diphtheria, tetanus, botulism and snake-bite poisoning.

The fact that pathogenic microbes stimulated antibody production in the blood had other important consequences. Richard Pfeiffer, a German bacteriologist, noted in 1895 that cholera and typhoid organisms clumped together and even disintegrated when placed in serum containing appropriate antibodies. This agglutination phenomenon led to the development of a diagnostic test for typhoid first used in 1896 by Fernand Widal of Paris. This was the beginning of serum diagnosis, which has since been employed in diagnosing a number of different communicable diseases. Another important development in this field was the complement fixation test, of which the principle was discovered in 1901 by Jules Bordet and Octave Gengou, and A. von Wassermann's modification of it as a test for syphilis in 1906.

The situation resulting from these discoveries was well described by Charles V. Chapin in 1910:

"We know now that direct contact with the sick, or with healthy carriers of disease germs, is an exceedingly frequent mode of transmission, and that infection by means of the air, or from infected articles, is not nearly as common as was formerly believed. We are now better able than ever before to attribute to water and milk their proper share in the distribution of infection. The recent discovery of the transmission of disease by insects gives us entirely new and most effective means of combating disease....The public health administrator is placed at great disadvantage

21

because he is obliged to base his acts on knowledge which is far from exact. The laboratory workers have accumulated a vast mass of quite exact data in regard to the causative relation of bacteria and protozoa to disease,...but there are many problems which the laboratory men cannot solve, and many others which they have failed to solve. The epidemiologist must study in the field the way in which disease is caused... [and] measure more carefully the relative importance of different sources of disease and different modes of infection."[6][7]

As Chapin indicates, with the identification of microorganisms responsible for particular communicable diseases and the clarification of their mode of action, the way was opened for the control of infectious diseases on a more specific, precise and rational basis. The early decades of the 20th century had a solid basis for primary prevention and control of a number of communicable diseases, but the question was which agencies and groups should be involved with and responsible for this task. The answer was formulated over several decades in terms of existing institutions and the creation of new ones, consistent with attitudes and beliefs prevalent in American society.

Inevitably the transformation of the United States from a rural agricultural nation into one predominantly industrial and urban was bound to have a profound effect on its political and other institutions. The resulting expansion of public functions was already evident during the later 19th century, but the full impact of this process in relation to health was not felt until well into the 20th century. The decades between 1900 and 1930 marked the first major period in the formulation of American social policy and legislation affecting health. To deal with the problems created by industrial expansion and economic insecurity, legislation was enacted for the protection of women and children, workmen's compensation schemes were inaugurated, interest was aroused in the financing, organization and provision of medical care, and the federal government tended more and more to assume responsibility for stimulating action by the states and localities.

One of the basic problems which concerned the pioneers of community action for disease prevention was the lack of adequate organization and administrative machinery. The civil service during the early nineteenth century was small in numbers, limited in function, and almost wholly recruited by patronage. A change from a haphazard to an efficient administration was essential for the development of a complicated urban, industrial society, capable of handling massive problems, among them dependency, disease and disability, and environmental hazards. The creation of the Metropolitan Board of Health in 1866 marks a turning point in this respect not only for New York City, but for the history of community health in the United States as a whole. The action taken in New York provided a model for others to follow, and new and effective health departments were established. Although an effort to create a national health department was only temporarily successful, by the end of the 19th century, a sound administrative basis had been created for the furtherance of community action to prevent and control disease. In fact, it was the provision of a stable structural base which made it relatively easy to incorporate new scientific knowledge into public health and medical practice.

As established in the 19th century, health departments were concerned essentially with the control of communicable diseases through environmental sanitation. The basic objective in abating sanitary nuisances was to prevent or to reduce morbidity and mortality caused by epidemics of cholera, yellow fever, typhus and enteric fevers. The occurrence of such diseases was generally considered due to environmental pollution resulting from lack of drainage, proper means for removing sewage and refuse, and inadequate provision of pure water. What was required was a program to identify cases of such diseases, to detect conditions likely to produce outbreaks, and to apply engineering skills to prevent or remove them. Within this context, the physician and the sanitary engineer were the chief figures in disease prevention, with the chemist providing analyses of water and food when required.

The health department with its relatively modest program was the major agency for disease prevention until bacteriology and immunology were brought to the United States in the 1880s. Although Americans contributed only in a limited degree to the growth of microbiological knowledge during this period, they were more alert than their European contemporaries to its practical applications. Out of this awareness there developed a new public health unit, the diagnostic laboratory for the application of bacteriology and immunology.

One of the earliest bacteriological laboratories in the United States was set up in 1887 by Joseph J. Kinyoun of the Marine Hospital Service on Staten Island in New York. In 1892 it was moved to Washington where a decade later it became the Hygienic Laboratory, the research arm of the Marine Hospital Service (Public Health Service, 1912), and later the nucleus of the present National Institutes of Health. Public health laboratories were also established in 1888 by Charles V. Chapin in Providence, R.I., and by Victor C. Vaughan for the Michigan State Health Department, primarily to analyze water and food.

It was in New York City, however, that the new knowledge of microbiology was first fully applied in the prevention and control of disease. Beginning in 1893 with a small diagnostic laboratory set up the previous year in response to the threat of a cholera invasion, William H. Park developed what amounted to an institute of applied microbiology in which work was done on diphtheria, tuberculosis, dysentery, penumonia, typhoid fever, scarlet fever, as well as numerous other diseases, and on the problems associated with them.

Establishment of public health laboratories by other local and state health departments followed rapidly after New York had set an example. It was clear that the application of microbiology held rich promise of usefulness in the control of communicable disease. Within a few years, almost every state and practically all large cities in the United States had established a diagnostic bacteriological laboratory. Through these laboratories, health departments to a considerable extent took over the task of diagnosing communicable diseases, and in order to control these diseases provided free biological products to doctors in practice and to public health officers. The growing influence of microbiology and the salient importance of the public health laboratory are clear from the establishment in 1899 by the American Public Health Association of a Section on Bacteriology and Chemistry (later the Laboratory Section). Upon its creation, almost 100 persons joined the Section.[68]

This event marked the emergence of a trend that developed with increased momentum in the first three decades of the present century, reflecting the widening scope and growing activism of the new public health based on expanding knowledge of disease prevention and health promotion. As a result, the American Public Health Association established the Section of Municipal Health Officers and the Vital Statistics Section in 1907-1908, the Sociological and Sanitary Engineering Sections in 1911, the Sections on Industrial Hygiene, and Food and Drugs in 1914 and 1917 respectively.[69] Four sections were created during the 1920s: Child Hygiene (1921), Health Education and Publicity (1922), Public Health Nursing (1923) and Epidemiology (1929).

These changes in the organizational structure of the American Public Health Association occurred in response to the consequences of a shift in the orientation of community health action, a major shift of attention from the physical aspects of the community to the people within it. Another indication of this change is evident in the American Medical Association during the same period. In 1900, the Section on State Medicine, which had been created in 1871, became the Section on Hygiene and Sanitary Science. It was renamed the Section on Preventive Medicine and Public Health in 1909, a title under which it continued until 1922 when it became the Section on Preventive and Industrial Medicine and Public Health.[70]

The meaning of these developments is that the problems of health which existed at the beginning of the century were being attacked by different groups using various strategies. One approach was through voluntary action. Such efforts by private individuals or groups have had an operational base in an organization developed specifically for the purpose of promoting an understanding of and action in the interest of handling certain community health problems. This organization, the voluntary health agency, is a distinctly modern institution which started out to provide health services of a kind that had not previously been available. It was a pioneer in putting to use for the common welfare new concepts and facts about health and disease, so that it should occasion little surprise to find the voluntary health agencies reflecting the social and medical tendencies of the period in which they arose and came to maturity, that is, the period from 1900 to 1930.

Historically, the voluntary health movement had two main roots. On the one hand, the voluntary agencies based their efforts on the concepts of health that had been developed and had gained acceptance by the end of the nineteenth century and during the early decades of the 20th. Important in this respect was the concept of the etiological specificity of disease, and almost equally important was the trend to specialization in medicine which led to a focus on organs or organ systems. On the other hand, these agencies developed out of efforts to grapple with poverty and privation, which revealed the destructive role of ill health in the lives of the poor, and the need for vigorous action to combat these conditions. In line with these origins, the voluntary health agencies have been concerned with furthering community health through education, by demonstrating ways of improving health services, by advancing related research and legislation, and perhaps as important as any of these by calling to public attention the existence of problems. The National Tuberculosis Association is the oldest agency of this type in the United States, and its evolution epitomizes the whole voluntary health movement and its relation to disease prevention.[71]

Before the 20th century, tuberculosis, like so many other communicable diseases, is believed to have exhibited a spontaneous ebb and flow in its prevalence and severity. From this viewpoint the experience with tuberculosis in the 19th century represents part of a long epidemic wave that reached its peak sometime around 1840 or 1850, and then slowly subsided. This experience was not limited to any single country, since records from western and central Europe, Great Britain, as well as the eastern United States reveal a similar pattern. The concept of tuberculosis as an infectious disease with a natural history must, however, also take into account the social factors involved in its causation. Tuberculosis is for the most part an endemic disease, protean in its manifestations, slow and insidious in its progress, selecting its victims from among those whose resistance is diminished, and thriving in deprived bodies. In this connection, it must be emphasized that living and working conditions are highly important in determining the tuberculosis experience of a population. Throughout the 19th century and beyond, the disease overwhelmingly affected urban communities. An urban community is a complicated structure within which no single factor operates alone to cause tuberculosis. As a result it is not easy to separate and weigh the interlocking, interdependent causative elements. One of the best studies of this problem was made by F.C.S. Bradbury, who, in 1930-31, investigated the high incidence of tuberculosis in the towns of Jarrow and Blaydon in England.[72] Bradbury concluded that the most important social factors were poverty, undernourishment, and overcrowding in dwellings. Poverty compels people to skimp on food, and to live in overcrowded rooms. It must be emphasized, however, that while poverty and tuberculosis can be closely linked in an ugly alliance, poor people need not become tubercular. Poverty, poor housing, overcrowding and malnutrition are important but secondary. The primary factor is the presence of an individual with an open case of the disease. In a community where tuberculosis is widely prevalent, most people from time to time come in contact with the pathogenic organism. On the whole, occasional fortuitous contacts are quite unimportant. Much more significant is close and regular contact over extended periods, as between husband and wife, parent and child, or other household members such as lodgers or servants. Contacts of this kind can also occur in places of employment, schools, or institutions such as mental hospitals. In such circumstances, lack of previous exposure to tuberculosis is an important predisposing factor. Among the millions of immigrants to the United States from 1880 to 1914 there were many from rural areas of Europe who came into contact with city dwellers, among whom tuberculosis had long been prevalent, under conditions favorable to the spread of the disease.

On March 4, 1882, Robert Koch announced his discovery of the tubercle bacillus as the etiologic agent of tuberculosis. The concept of tuberculosis as a disease entity, originally set up on purely clinical and pathological-anatomical grounds, was now confirmed by bacteriological evidence. The implications of this discovery for community action were soon recognized in Great Britain, France and several other European countries, nor did the United States remain uninfluenced by these developments. As early as 1899, a report prepared by Hermann M. Biggs, J. Mitchell Prudden and H.P. Loomis, consulting pathologists to the New York City Health Department, emphasized the preventability of tuberculosis, and recommended surveillance of the disease by the department as well as education of the public concerning its nature. In 1894 the department began to require reporting of cases of tuberculosis by institutions, and in 1897 reporting by physicians. Similar efforts were undertaken at about the same time by local health officers and physicians in other communities.

Up to this point, however, the war against tuberculosis was a matter for the professional. The mobilization of the forces of the community for the control of a disease was first undertaken in the United States during the same decade. The discovery of the potentialities of broad community organization as a means of controlling disease was to have far-reaching significance for the entire community health program. This novel and pregnant conception was introduced by the pioneers of the anti-tuberculosis movement, particularly the Philadelphia physician Lawrence F. Flick and his associates, who organized the Pennsylvania Society for the Prevention of Tuberculosis in 1892, After the passage of a decade this example was followed elsewhere in the United States, so that by the beginning of 1904 twenty-three state and local societies had been formed. Recognition of the need for a national organization led to the formation in June 1904 of the National Association for the Study and Prevention of Tuberculosis. (In 1918 the name was changed to the National Tuberculosis Association).[73]

By this time, the situation with respect to preventive action was considerably clarified. Initial attempts to produce active or passive immunization had failed, nor had any specific therapy been developed. Koch's announcement in 1890 of a preparation from tubercle bacilli as a curative and preventive agent for tuberculosis soon led to disappointment when experience showed that it was useless and even dangerous. There was agreement, however, on the value of tuberculin, as Koch's preparation was called, for diagnosis, and it remained in use for this purpose.[74] Nevertheless, this immunological limitation was counterbalanced by increasing knowledge of the characteristics of the causal agent, and of the routes by which it was transmitted. Studies by G. Cornet, C. Flügge and others showed that tubercle bacilli were transmitted through infected sputum either as droplets expelled by coughing or as dust particles after expectorated sputum had dried. Even though these views were only partly correct, they emphasized the danger of careless expectoration of sputum, e.g. on floors or into handkerchiefs, and provided a rationale for preventive measures.[75]

Central to the prevention of tuberculosis was avoidance of exposure to infection, thus interrupting the chain of transmission. This principle, interruption of transmission by separating the affected individuals from others, and thus rendering them ineffective as sources of the pathogenic microbe, was not new. Introduced in Europe during the Middle Ages, initially to combat leprosy and then plague, it had given rise to an important tool of primary prevention, the practice of quarantine. Owing to ignorance or inadequate knowledge of the etiology and epidemiology of communicable diseases, however, quarantine measures were of only questionable effectiveness until the beginning of the 20th century.[76] The microbiological discoveries made it possible for health authorities to act with greater discrimination in carrying out preventive procedures. By establishing the incubation period in a given disease, the number of days required for isolation could be set more exactly. Similarly, by showing how water or food transmitted disease under given conditions, control measures could be undertaken more effectively. The first decade of the 20th century thus had a solid, expanding scientific basis for the control of a number of communicable diseases, and throughout succeeding decades up to the present advances in these terms have continued.

Methods and techniques have naturally varied for different diseases. In the case of tuberculosis, practical techniques for staining tubercle bacilli were developed in 1882 by Paul Ehrlich and F. Ziehl, thus making it possible to identify the organism in sputum and other materials.[77] The practical use of tuberculin for diagnosis was made possible by the skin test introduced by Clemens von Pirquet in 1907. A year later, G. Mantoux described the intradermal test which then became standard practice.[78] Although the use of x-rays, including fluoroscopy, was discussed at the Sixth International Congress on Tuberculosis which met in 1908 in Washington, D.C., radiography was first employed systematically as a diagnostic tool in 1917 in the Framingham Community Health and Tuberculosis Demonstration.[79]

The strategy for an attack on tuberculosis, aimed at its prevention, developed within the context described above. A specific biologic enemy was known, the tubercle bacillus, as were its social allies that fostered the spread of the disease: depressed living standards, poor, overcrowded housing, insanitary and unhealthful conditions at work, undernourishment, and precarious economic circumstances, in fact all the problems that brought into being the movement for social betterment. The strategy employed to fight tuberculosis may be characterized as socio-medical. In order to know the extent of the problem, compulsory reporting of cases of tuberculosis was necessary. Physicians and hospitals caring for such patients were to register them with the appropriate health agency, a municipal or county health department. To dispel ignorance and fear of the disease, and to achieve support for measures of compulsion, the general public had to be informed about its nature, transmission, and means of control. Education was also required for patients and their families, particularly with respect to personal habits and hygiene. Furthermore, sanatoria were needed for the isolation and care of tuberculous patients, and clinics to examine those who had had contact with active cases or who were suspected of having the disease. Finally, to obtain legislation establishing such facilities and to secure the removal of the social evils contributing to the propagation of tuberculosis, public support had to be rallied and effectively organized.

The campaign against tuberculosis was undertaken by physicians, social workers and public spirited citizens in a crusading spirit, and it is certainly not a matter of chance that military terms pervade the publicity employed by the anti-tuberculosis movement. At first the chief aims were early discovery and isolation of cases so as to prevent the spread of infection, to strike at the germ by finding and treating the early case. These aims were pursued as vigorously as possible, but it gradually became clear that matters were not so simple. Findings that early infection was widespread among urban inhabitants, and that most infected individuals did not develop recognizable disease led to an increased emphasis on environmental factors involving public and personal hygiene, including clean streets, fresh air, proper nutrition, pure food and personal cleanliness, what Ida M. Cannon called the "hygienic gospel."[80]

The impact of the environmental emphasis ramified in several directions and affected prevention of other diseases, particularly those of infancy and childhood. As Allen K. Krause observed in 1927, "All of us like to grow eloquent anent the revolution wrought by tuberculosis propaganda in the sleeping habits of a nation; how in a few short years a people, holding age-long fears of the dangers of night air to health, opened its bedroom windows and accustomed itself to a restorative that must, in the large, be having incalculable effects for good." A second beneficial consequence which he noted derived from

"the broader results of the supervision of cattle and of milk supplies. Perhaps the close watch on herds and dairies and the pasteurization of city milk would have come as soon and as effectively without the ghost of consumption . . . to spur them on. But one must doubt it; just as one must doubt whether thousands of children would be alive today had not their milk, in their babyhood and later, been treated for the germs of tuberculosis, and in the process cleansed of other germs of far less tenacity of life yet of greater immediate virulence."[81]

One facet of the tuberculosis problem to which Krause alluded, and which was not understood until the 20th century, was the relation of tuberculosis in cattle to the disease in man. Cases of tuberculous glands and joints, which were common in earlier periods and in the earlier years of this century, were most often due to milk contaminated with the bovine strain of the tubercle bacillus. Koch believed that all tubercle bacilli, whether in man or other mammals, were the same. In 1896, however, Theobald Smith, at the Bureau of Animal Husbandry, demonstrated the existence of two different strains and opened up the way to clarify human infection with bovine tubercle bacilli. In 1883, O. Bollinger and his associates at the Munich Pathological Institute showed that milk from a tuberculous cow when injected into a guinea pig killed it in a few weeks, and other guinea pigs treated similarly with secretions and tissues of infected cows showed lesions with tubercle bacilli. In 1902-04, M.P. Ravenel, at the Henry Phipps Institute in Philadelphia, pointed out the pathogenicity of bovine tubercle bacilli in man and emphasized the danger of transmitting tuberculosis from cattle to human beings. The matter was finally settled by the definitive report of William H. Park and Charles Krumwiede in 1912, who demonstrated that a large proportion of tuberculosis in children, intestinal tuberculosis and tuberculosis of the glands of the neck, was due to ingestion of contaminated milk.[82]

Since bovine tuberculosis caused about one fifth to a quarter of the cases in infants and children, it was evident that bovine tubercle bacilli played a significant role in the etiology of childhood tuberculosis, and that prevention had to deal with the bovine source by breaking the chain of transmission. This aim could be achieved in two ways, by eliminating bovine tuberculosis in cattle, and by pasteurizing milk. Both approaches were pursued. Although dairy inspection had begun in Newark, New Jersey, as early as 1882, and pasteurization about a decade later, the movement was slow. Chicago enacted a compulsory pasteurization ordinance in 1909, the first such law in the United

States.[83] New York followed in 1910. Jordan estimated that in 1910 about 50 percent of the total milk supply of Boston was pasteurized, but there was no health department regulation covering the practice. In 1912, Rosenau noted that "other cities and states appear backward in promulgating laws and regulations upon the subject of pasteurization." Nonetheless, the situation was improving for "the amount of pasteurized milk in most of our large cities is showing a steady increase."[84] It was not until the 1930s, however, that the full effects were felt. By that time, for example, 91 percent of the milk consumed in the twin cities of Minneapolis and St. Paul was pasteurized.[85] In Chicago, despite the 1909 ordinance, opposition from dairy interests prevented the tuberculin testing of herds outside the city until 1925, when the Chicago health commissioner proposed to bar all milk from untested cattle. In a dramatic clash between state and city, Chicago emerged victorious and the situation improved thereafter. By the middle 1940s, according to a survey by the U.S. Public Health Service, all milk consumed in Chicago was pasteurized.[86]

The elimination of bovine tuberculosis by killing tuberculous animals and recompensing the owners was started in 1917 as a national program under the Department of Agriculture. By employing systematic tuberculin testing, prompt slaughtering of infected animals, thorough disinfection and appropriate procedures for the movement of cattle, the reactor rate of tested cattle fell from 4.9 percent in 1918 to 0.08 percent in 1965.[87]

The campaign to eradicate bovine tuberculosis, particularly through the increasing practice of pasteurization, had a significant impact on the transmission of other communicable diseases. Milk as a vehicle for the transmission of typhoid fever had first been incriminated in 1857 by William Taylor in England, but not until 1881 was attention first clearly directed to the danger of the spread of epidemic diseases by milk. That year, at the International Medical Congress in London, Ernest Hart reported 50 epidemics of typhoid fever, 15 epidemics of scarlet fever, and four epidemics of diphtheria attributed to this cause. In 1909, the U.S. Public Health Service issued its famous Bulletin 56, which listed 500 outbreaks of milkborne disease between 1880 and 1907. These epidemics were noted when they were severe, as in Boston between 1907 and 1911 when the city had five milk-borne outbreaks (diphtheria, scarlet fever, typhoid fever, and "tonsillitis", probably streptococcal sore throat). But as Rosenau pointed out in 1912, these outbreaks were not always reported because "they are becoming 'twice-told tales'."[88] Furthermore, many an infant was sent to an early grave through drinking contaminated milk. Infantile diarrhea (summer complaint, cholera infantum) practically controlled the curve of infant mortality, and exhibited a high seasonal prevalence every summer. Studies by William H. Park and L. Emmett Holt, the eminent pediatrician, clearly showed that during hot weather the kind of milk fed to infants influenced the amount of illness to which they were sub-

30

ject and their mortality. As we shall see shortly, the provision of pure milk was a very important factor in the reduction of infant mortality.

Obviously, a preventive measure such as pasteurization intended to provide uncontaminated milk was an attack not on one disease or one health problem, but rather on several. Such measures, of which the effects ramify in several directions, can reinforce the action of other procedures and approaches for combating specific diseases or problems. Consequences of this kind, whether intended or not, may be termed *synergistic preventive effects,* or perhaps broad spectrum prevention. For example, attention to tuberculosis among industrial workers tended to reinforce the movement to improve conditions in factories and workshops for all workers.[89] The principle of synergistic prevention is important in endeavoring to understand the evolution of disease and health problems that are complex in origin and have no simple solutions, as for example tuberculosis, venereal diseases, and the diseases associated with infancy.

In bovine tuberculosis, the pathogenic organism could be attacked directly by destroying the infected host or by treating the product, milk, so as to render it safe for consumption. These methods could be applied because the force of law eventually coincided with the economic interests of the cattle and the dairy industries. Since these methods were inapplicable to human beings, the alternative was to find the early case, segregate the patient in a sanatorium or by teaching the patient and the family to observe strict hygienic practices so as to prevent transmission, and to follow-up the contacts. These aims were implemented through programs of case-finding, and by establishing diagnostic clinics and sanatoria. By the 1920s, it had been recognized in principle that tuberculosis prevention and control was a governmental responsibility exercised at the municipal, county and state levels.[90] The federal government did not become actively involved in the administrative control of tuberculosis until 1944, despite some action by Surgeon-General Parran shortly after Pearl Harbor.[91] However, the implementation of the principle left much to be desired. A survey by the Public Health service in 1923 of activities in 100 municipalities led to the conclusion that the diagnostic clinics were insufficient in number and inefficiently administered. Furthermore, in most states the number of sanatorium beds was wholly inadequate to meet the needs. In fact, some cities and counties did not have half enough beds.[92] Not only were the facilities for diagnosed cases inadequate, but physicians were limited in their ability to detect early tuberculosis by the available diagnostic methods. This was also a transitional period in medical education, a period in which there were numerous physicians who had not been properly taught to recognize manifestations of early pulmonary tuberculosis. There were still others whose approach was limited by their socio-economic views. In Muncie, Indiana, for example, the local Anti-tuberculosis Association maintained a weekly chest clinic to which physicians from the County Medical Society donated their services with the proviso that the clinic should be available only to those too poor to pay privately.[93] Until the early 1930s x-rays were used unsystematically and sporadically for the detection of early tuberculosis. Mass survey techniques had not yet been developed. With the introduction of cheap paper films around 1931 and miniature photo-roentgen films after 1936, low cost mass chest x-ray surveys became possible.[94] Such surveys became an important function of health departments, another indication that official health agencies were taking over the task of controlling tuberculosis. Assistance was given to many communities by the U.S. Public Health Service. Acceptance of mass x-ray services by labor unions, business executives, and the general public led to surveys of occupational groups, selected community groups considered to be at high risk, and after World War II, from about 1946 to 1953, to a number of large city surveys. During this period chest x-ray programs were started in general hospitals on all admissions and proved productive.[95] During the same period three chemotherapeutic agents were introduced, streptomycin in 1947, para-aminosalicylic acid in 1949, and isonazid in 1952 with the result that the pattern of tuberculosis prevention and control began to change markedly. Sanatoria and special hospitals closed since no prolonged stays in institutions were required, tuberculosis specialists disappeared or no longer limited their work to the disease, the voluntary associations saw the handwriting on the wall and expanded their scope to include respiratory diseases, and health departments rearranged their priorities so that activities concerned with tuberculosis were downgraded. The amount of tuberculosis in the United States declined but the disease did not disappear.

What had happened to the disease over the past 75 years? In 1900, on the basis of census data for the preceding decade, it became apparent that the general death rate per 1000 had dropped from 19.6 in 1890 to 17.8 in 1900, but that the decline for tuberculosis from 2.4 to 2.0 was more rapid. This had occurred during a period when more and more people were moving into cities where tuberculosis was a major problem, a point emphasized by Krause in 1927.[96] Indeed, by 1900 tuberculosis had already retreated to second place among the leading causes of death, a fact which was mildly encouraging to those bent on attacking it.[97] From this point to the present, mortality has declined constantly and sometimes rapidly, though the number of new active cases has dropped more slowly. The tuberculosis death rate declined relatively slowly until 1918-1919. Between 1918 and 1921 there was a sharp drop, and thereafter until the mid-1940s the decline accelerated. From 1918 to 1921 the tuberculosis death rate declined by one-third, from 149.8 to 97.6, and the question may be raised whether this was a consequence of the influenza pandemic of 1918. Though death rates for influenza were higher among those with pulmonary tuberculosis than among the general population, Allen K. Krause, an astute student of the problem, considered this factor as relatively minor though he did admit that it might have had some effect on the death rates.[98] Be that as it may, the dramatic decrease from 33.5 in 1946 to 9.1 in 1955 was undoubtedly due to the introduction of chemotherapy in the former year. By 1966 the mortality rate had declined to 3.9.

The dropping mortality and the slower decline in new active cases represent a slow retreat before a prolonged and sustained attack on the disease, chiefly the pulmonary form. This must not be taken to mean, however, that the decline of tuberculosis morbidity and mortality can be attributed alone to the activities of the anti-tuberculosis movement. The decline of tuberculosis between 1900 and the present can be seen as the expression, in slow motion, of an evolving biosocial process, perhaps best described by Wade H. Frost's concept of biological attrition.[99] He recognized that the risk of infection, morbidity and mortality in a disease of slow evolution and long duration such as tuberculosis required investigation over an extended period:

> "For tuberculosis . . . we cannot assume that the risk with which we are concerned is concentrated within the year or even the decade following the establishment of the known exposure. It may, perhaps, be manifested by excessive morbidity and mortality in any subsequent period of life. Hence, observation of the exposed group must extend over a sufficient number of years to define the rates of morbidity and mortality prevailing in successive periods throughout the usual span of life."[100]

This process results from the interaction of the biological characteristics of the tubercle bacillus and of the human host with environmental factors in a dynamic equilibrium. Naturally such a balance is unstable and can be upset by unfavorable environmental conditions such as those produced by wars or other major social disruptions. Tuberculosis flared up in Europe during World War I and again during the Second World War. During the post-war period with a return to more normal conditions, the situation improved and tuberculosis continued to decline. The experience of Great Britain during World War II is striking. After a rise of about 11 percent in the overall tuberculosis mortality during 1940 and 1941, the downward trend of the prewar period was resumed in 1942 and continued without further interruption.[101] This experience was undoubtedly influenced by the considerable reduction in the number of cases between 1914 and 1939, but a very important factor was the policy of the British government to see that all essential nutrients should be equally available to everyone to an extent necessary for the maintenance of health. Certain foods such as margarine and flour were fortified by the addition of vitamins (A and D) and minerals (calcium). On the other hand, the poor experience of Germany and Austria with respect to tuberculosis at the end of World War I and during the immediate post-war years was due in considerable measure to the hunger and privation resulting from the blockade imposed by the Allies, reinforced by the subsequent inflation. Mortality rates per 100,000 in Germany increased from 1921 through 1923, then resumed a downward trend again in 1924 with the reestablishment of more stable economic and social conditions. Interestingly enough, the highest rate reached during the immediate post-war period, 147 per 100,000 in 1923, still remained below the rate of 158 in 1911. In fact, by 1926 the mortality rate had declined to 98 per 100,000.[102] The significance of these examples is clearly indicated by Krause's insistence in 1918 that emphasis be "laid on the behavior of the human being and not on the bacillus."[103]

What this means is that the prevention and control of tuberculosis have been achieved by taking action to tip the balance in favor of actual and potential human hosts. Frost saw this in 1937 when he wrote,

"it is a fair inference that in this country as a whole we have already reached the stage at which the biological balance is against the survival of the tubercle bacillus, for year by year the mortality from tuberculosis is decreasing . . . This means that under present conditions of human resistance and environment the tubercle bacillus is losing ground, and that the eventual eradication of tuberculosis requires only that the present balance against it be maintained."[104]

Although Frost's postulation of the eventual eradication of tuberculosis is still to be realized, actions concerned with other problems as well as those intended to combat tuberculosis have tended to create an ever more unfavorable situation for the pathogenic organism.

The outbreak of the First World War interrupted the great Atlantic migration which since the 1880s had brought millions of Europeans to the United States where they settled largely in urban centers. The cessation of immigration during the war years and the restrictive legislation of 1921 and 1924 were undoubtedly important factors in changing the circumstances of the foreign born. As the flow of new immigrants was cut down to a trickle, the foreign born and even more so their children tended to improve their mode of life under the influence of economic and educational factors.[105] As they moved up the economic ladder, even if only moderately, there was an increasing tendency to move out of the areas of initial settlement into sections with better housing. Between 1920 and 1930 a growing trend appeared toward less clustering of the foreign born in ethnic neighborhoods. Many of those involved in this process of change were younger persons of the native-born generation, with a greater earning capacity and thus able to afford a higher standard of living. Although the depression of the 1930s retarded these tendencies, they revived toward the end of the decade coincident with the outbreak of World War II and continued after the war.

During the same period, housing was being improved. By 1937, central heating, hot and cold running water, and interior installed toilets and baths were commonplace essentials in millions of houses. Nonetheless, such advances were uneven; overcrowding in houses and living conditions conducive to ill health were still present. A comprehensive survey of housing in 64 cities conducted in 1934 revealed that even by moderate standards 15.6 percent of the houses were overcrowded. Almost one-fifth had no private indoor toilets and about one-quarter were without installed bathing facilities. All in all, approximately four million urban American families were still without what in 1937 were termed "modern improvements"—running water, indoor private toilets and baths. In addition, there were possibly twice that number in rural areas.[106]

As the disease declined, living conditions improved though not equally in all segments of communities, even when the inhabitants were of the same ethnic stock.[107] Unfavorable conditions persisted in the socially remote sectors where living standards were low, for example, among Negroes in urban centers, the majority of whom lived on the lowest economic level, affected not only by poor housing but also by inadequate nutrition and lack of other basic necessities.[108] The role of nutrition as a probable factor in the evolution of tuberculosis has already been mentioned, but it must also be emphasized that special attention began to be given to the nutritional status of the population between the two World Wars. The necessity to safeguard health while conserving food during the First World War led to the production of increased supplies of protective foods and a growing recognition of their value. Improved methods of producing and distributing perishable foods made protective foods more easily available in urban communities. Furthermore, the development of more effective advertising and merchandising methods for fruits, vegetables, milk and other products led to their increased use. The growth of chain stores, cafeterias and restaurants also facilitated the distribution of perishable food to consumers. At the same time, in the 1920s, interest in improving the nutrition of children and of mothers during the childbearing period was furthered by the Maternal and Infancy Act. Attention to nutrition was further stimulated bya the world economic crisis of 1929-1936, when widespread malnutrition followed on the heels of mass unemployment, as well as by the special needs of the Second World War with its attendant food shortages, rationing, and the necessity for protecting workers in industry, as well as women and children. After 1935, the Federal Surplus Commodities Corporation provided food for school lunches, and by the end of 1938, 45 states and the District of Columbia were participating in this activity. In May 1939, the Food Stamp Plan was inaugurated to supply families on relief and those with low incomes with food. In 1940 and 1941, a total of $235,000,000 was available for the distribution of agricultural surpluses through the stamp plan, through relief agencies, and for school lunches. These activities undoubtedly had a beneficial effect on the nutritional status of a large segment of the American population, thus contributing to the continuing decline of tuberculosis.[109]

The significance of these factors was already noted by Frost in 1937:

"Probably nothing has been more influential in bringing about the decline of tuberculosis than progressive improvement in the social order as a whole; and nothing, perhaps, is more essential to the further effective control of the disease than to hold up, and so far as possible to improve the standards of living of the lower economic strata . . . It is probable that one of the most important factors in the decline of tuberculosis has been progressively increasing human resistance, due to the influence of selective mortality and to environmental improvements such as better nutrition and relief from physical stress tending to raise what may be called nonspecific resistance."[110]

Discussing the great increase in tuberculosis in Europe after the Second World War, Johannes Holm made the same point as Frost but he added another significant factor. According to Holm, the marked rise was due to malnutrition which lowered resistance; overcrowded living conditions in the large cities, and a low standard of personal hygiene because facilities for cleanliness and hygiene were nonexistent, thus enabling tubercle bacilli to appear, *and* the disorganization of the anti-tuberculosis program in many European countries.[111]

The implication of Holm's analysis is that a fundamental element in any practical program of disease prevention is the existence of an organized institutional framework within which it can be implemented. If such a structured context does not exist, or is inadequate, or is disrupted as happened in Europe, it is difficult if not impossible to carry out a coherent and consistent preventive program. In fact, this is one of the difficulties in the United States today with respect to cardiovascular disease, neoplasms, and a number of other health problems to be discussed below. To put the matter in another way, one reason why the socioeconomic conditions of the Depression did not materially affect the continuing decline of tuberculosis was the existence of a well developed preventive program which was being carried out within a coherent institutional arrangement comprising official health agencies, voluntary organizations and medical practitioners. The relationship between these elements has altered over the years. Tuberculosis control became a major component of the community health program by the 1920s, and the health department, though working in cooperation with voluntary tuberculosis groups and practitioners, acquired a central role. Its activities included reporting and registration, case finding, clinical, x-ray and laboratory services, nursing service, health education and institutional care, and required the employment of professional and technical personnel, such as physicians, nurses, bacteriologists, x-ray and laboratory technicians as well as others.[112] As tuberculosis progressively declined, the control program has necessarily been readjusted, and has also changed in direction, influenced considerably by chemoprophylaxis and chemotherapy.

Tuberculosis has been discussed in some detail because it provides a model of a disease resulting from a complex interaction of biological, socio-economic and cultural factors. Though a specific etiologic agent has been known for almost a hundred years, a high degree of prevention and control has not been achieved by a frontal attack on the organism, but by drying up the sources of infection through isolation of patients, pasteurization of milk, by reducing overcrowding in dwellings, improving nutrition, and in general raising living standards and making it possible for people to maintain them by increasing their economic resources. These tactical moves were made possible by efforts to educate the general public to the nature of the disease, to win over community leaders and public officials to support necessary measures, to improve the quality of medical education and practice with respect to tuberculosis, and to provide the services required to restore the patient to community life.

The strategy and tactics developed in dealing with the prevention and control of tuberculosis have in general also been used in handling other complex health problems. The idea of organizing to control a specific disease or a group of disorders, and of enlisting community support and action through an organized and systematic campaign of public education soon spread to other fields.[113] In 1905 Dr. Prince A. Morrow organized the Society for Social and Moral Prophylaxis to deal with the prevention and treatment of venereal diseases. Similar societies were formed in 11 States, and by 1910 these were united in the American Federation for Sex Hygiene, which in 1914 joined with the American Vigilance Association to form the American Social Hygiene Association. The time was propitious and the need for action was apparent. The concept of sin and the moral sanction with which Western society, particularly in England and America, surrounded sex relations exerted an unfortunate influence on the attitudes of the medical profession as well as of the lay public to practitioners devoting themselves to diseases of the genito-urinary organs. The social disapprobation which was the lot of the unfortunate victims of syphilis and gonorrhea was extended in greater or lesser degree to the physicians to whom they turned for treatment. The result was that a great many refused to treat such patients in their private practice so as to avoid being known as a "clap doctor." Since clinics or hospital facilities were often unavailable, these patients were forced into the hands of unscrupulous practitioners and quacks.[114] These attitudes were associated with the social hypocrisy of ignoring sexual activity and its consequences, while maintaining a double standard regulating relations between the sexes, for the most part to the disadvantage of women. Nevertheless, the erosion of these social attitudes had begun in the period before the First World War. In 1912, a Philadelphia physician, Robert N. Wilson, said: "It seems incredible that up to the present syphilis and gonococcus infection are, officially speaking, nonexistent, and that as far as the national, and to a greater extent the municipal, authorities are concerned, are deserving only of contempt or complete disregard."[115] This assertion seems to be borne out by findings in 227 cities survey in 1913.[116] Only seven required reporting of venereal diseases, four had free clinics for such patients, and only three provided hospital care for serious cases. Forty-six cities did provide free laboratory diagnostic facilities for syphilis, but this was related to the inspection of prostitutes which was still employed as a significant control measure.

During this period, accurate knowledge and some effective means for dealing with problems associated with gonorrhea and syphilis were already available. As previously mentioned, Albert Neisser had described the gonococcus in 1879 and demonstrated its presence in ophthalmia neonatorum. Then, in 1884, the obstetrician K.S.F. Credé, emphasizing that infection occurred during the infant's passage through the birth canal, found that the resulting gonorrheal ophthalmia could be prevented by instilling a drop of 2 percent silver nitrate in each eye immediately after birth.[117] All that was required was to train obstetricians and midwives to carry out the requisite procedure.

Nevertheless, in the United States progress was slow due largely to the poor quality of obstetrical care provided to many women. Nor had public authorities been active in improving the situation. During this period 1906-1911, this prophylactic measure was required in only one state. Another indication of the situation is the finding among a group of children in schools for the blind surveyed in 1907 that 28.2 percent suffered from blindness due to gonorrheal ophthalmia. By 1923, however, the situation was improving. At that time, 81 cities required the routine use of silver nitrate prophylaxis, and 84 cities required reporting of cases. Yet these data indicate a continuing need for improvement since only in 41 cities were any records kept of reported cases of ophthalmia neonatorum or of the treatment given. However, as states and municipalities enacted legislation requiring the use of silver nitrate drops in the eyes of newborns, and as obstetrical practice improved, the incidence and prevalence declined progressively. By 1936-1941, 46 states required preventive action, and the percentage of admissions to schools for the blind due to ophthalmia neonatorum had dropped to 7.4 percent. By 1954-1955, this percent declined to 0.1, and in 1958-1959 the incidence of gonorrheal ophthalmia was 0.3 percent.[118]

This development was the consequence of several interacting factors operating over the past 60 years. First, a specific agent was known to cause ophthalmia neonatorum, and the source of infection was also known. Secondly, a simple, specific means of prevention was available. Thirdly, the newborn baby could not affect its situation by its behavior. Moreover, more and more deliveries were taking place in hospitals where prophylaxis could be practised routinely. This situation was reinforced by a fourth factor, the influence exerted on public opinion, among legislators and public officials, and on the medical profession by the movements to improve the health of infants and

38

children, and to prevent venereal diseases and their complications.

The interaction of these factors made it possible to deal with gonorrheal ophthalmia, even though there was no satisfactory means for the primary prevention of gonorrhea in sexually mature men and women, except by avoidance of exposure through continence or the use of the condom, or by medical prophylaxis which could be used effectively with individuals under strict discipline as in the army or navy. In 1937, the introduction of the sulfonamides seemed to provide a therapy which would lessen the possibility of transmission, but the appearance of drug resistant strains soon scotched this hope. Nor did the subsequent appearance of penicillin improve the situation very much. In point of fact, gonorrhea has not been effectively prevented or controlled in the United States. A consideration of the past 35 years finds the number of cases reported to the Public Health Service rising from a low of 193,468 in 1941 to a peak of 400,639 in 1947. Thereafter the number of cases declined to 216,448 in 1957, after which a rise began which has far exceeded the high point of 1947. In 1970, 600,072 civilian cases were reported. The rates per 100,000 population have varied accordingly.[119] Since reporting of cases remains poor, particularly those treated by private practitioners, these figures very likely represent only the tip of an iceberg.[120] An estimated one million cases were believed to have been unreported in 1970.

Given the widespread and increasing prevalence of gonorrhea, it is not surprising to find a recrudescence of cases of ophthalmia neonatorum, a situation in which, even though the numbers so far have been small, the problem of prophylaxis has been reconsidered. The reappearance of gonorrheal ophthalmia in newborns is due not only to the wide prevalence of gonorrhea, but has been favored also by additional factors. As has already been emphasized, all forms of prevention must be seen in their ecological contexts where various factors may facilitate or hinder their effectiveness.

Sometimes professional shortsightedness leads physicians to overlook the wider context of a preventive measure and to neglect or drop it because the condition at which it is aimed is no longer prevalent, and the benefits are believed to be outweighed by alleged harmful effects. In 1957, after silver nitrate prophylaxis was discontinued at the Sloane Hospital for women, a 15-fold increase in cases of gonorrheal ophthalmia among newborns occurred over the subsequent seven-month period. Similarly, the disease has reappeared in Glasgow where prophylaxis was discontinued several years ago.[121]

Another, more important factor is the increased incidence of gonorrhea in adolescents and young adults, which provides a large asymptomatic reservoir among females. Surveys of gonorrhea among pregnant women in clinics show an incidence of about 6 percent, while findings among patients in private practice are also quite high.[122] Many of these women harbor subclinical infections. These findings and their implications have brought in their wake an increased emphasis on silver nitrate prophylaxis, and an identification of infection in pregnant women leading to prompt adequate treatment. Forty years ago, Lehrfeld expressed the view that silver nitrate prophylaxis was essentially secondary prevention, noting that

> "The fundamental principles of all public health measures deal with the control of disease at its source. Yet in ophthalmia neonatorum all health officers are content to wait until the infant has been exposed to the disease and place full reliance on the prevention after exposure."[123]

Diagnosis and treatment of infection in the gravid woman, according to Lehrfeld, would be a primary preventive approach since it would be aimed at the source. This point of view expresses a basic principle of preventive medicine, and in a clinic or hospital situation with current methods of diagnosis and therapy would appear to offer a greater chance of success than was the case in 1935. Moreover, it might contribute toward interruption of the chain of transmission among adults. Nevertheless, in the light of current attitudes toward sexual activity, associated among some groups with poor hygienic practices and antagonism to health agencies, both treatment of the mother where possible and routine use of silver nitrate prophylaxis for the newborn seem necessary.[124]

The prevention of congenital syphilis has had an analogous development. Views on the causation, diagnosis and treatment of syphilis were illuminated and altered during the first decade of the century by the identification of a specific etiologic agent, the *Spirochaeta pallida* in 1905, and by the introduction of the Wassermann test in 1906, as well as the use of the chemotherapeutic agent salvarsan in 1910.[125] Congenital syphilis and its consequences for morbidity and mortality among infants also began to engage professional and public attention about this time both in the United States and Europe.[126] From 1900 almost to 1940 the death rate from syphilis was particularly high during the first year of life. The highest death rate for syphilis among infants under one year of age in the United States was 134.8 per 100,000 population during 1916. By 1923 the rate declined to 86.5, and then fluctuated between 77 and 87 per 100,000 from 1924 through 1937. Thereafter the deaths from syphilis in children under one year of age dropped sharply from 1300 deaths in 1939 to 25 in 1965, as did the rates per 100,000 live births, from 57.4 to 0.7.[127] For all practical purposes, syphilis has disappeared as a cause of infant mortality. The basic reason for this decline was the prevention of congenital syphilis by treating infected pregnant women during the prenatal period, and by finding and treating infants with congenital syphilis. In short, the strategy was primarily to attack the source of the problem, precisely the approach proposed for the prevention of gonococcal ophthalmia in newborns. But syphilis could be detected much more precisely through serologic testing and this tool began to be applied together with chemotherapy soon after 1910.

Although the need to deal with the problem of congenital syphilis by means of antenatal prophylaxis and early treatment was recognized before 1910, in practice there was no effective therapy except the use of mercury in one form or another.[128] Initially, Ehrlich warned against the use of salvarsan for the treatment of syphilitic gravid women, but within five years after its introduction a number of French, Scandinavian and German physicians had demonstrated its effectiveness in preventing syphilitic infection of the newborn.[129]

In the United States, Urquhart had suggested as early as 1909 that "the application of Wassermann's[sic] reaction would be of very practical value" in selecting a wet-nurse for a healthy infant.[130] Several years later, in 1916, J. Whitridge Williams instituted a routine Wassermann test on all women attending the prenatal clinic at the Johns Hopkins Hospital. An analysis of 700 fetal deaths among 10,000 consecutive deliveries in the obstetrical service of the Hospital had revealed that 26 percent were due to syphilis, and Williams became convinced "that the only way in which the problem could be approached with any hope of effective solution was by determining the Wassermann reaction in every pregnant woman who registered in the dispensary, and subjecting her to intensive treatment whenever it was positive."[131] The results at Johns Hopkins and at other institutions soon demonstrated the value of this approach, and by the mid 1920s it had been adopted as the best way to prevent congenital lues.[132] The practice was reinforced by legislative enactments requiring a serologic test for syphilis for pregnant women before or after delivery. In 1938 Rhode Island enacted the first state law requiring a prenatal blood test for pregnant women. By 1964, 42 states had such a legal requirement.[133] Despite the very marked drop in reported cases of congenital syphilis in the past 30 years, since 1957 there has been an increase among newborns. The reported incidence has risen from 0.4 cases per 10,000 live births in 1957 to 1.0 in 1966. This rise parallels the rising incidence of primary and secondary cases for females, from 2.6 cases per 100,000 population in 1957 to 8.8 in 1966.[134] These infections occur overwhelmingly among infants whose mothers have had inadequate or no prenatal care and who deliver at home, or who are delivered at a hospital where they first receive medical attention. This seems to parallel the situation with respect to gonococcal ophthalmia neonatorum.

Central to the prevention of these infections is organized prenatal care, which developed out of a desire to reduce infant mortality by teaching mothers how to feed and care for their babies, and out of a recognition that the health of the mother in pregnancy influenced the condition of her

41

unborn child. In 1909, addressing the Conference on Prevention of Infant Mortality in New Haven, C.-E.A. Winslow asserted that "Nowhere is the necessity for joining these two forces Prevention and Education. . . more urgent than in the campaign against infant mortality. . . The systematic education of mothers must be the key-note of any really successful campaign against infant mortality."[135]

Williams recognized that prevention of fetal or infant death was a socio-medical problem which required the cooperation of patient and physician. The achievement of this aim presupposed

"not only first-rate obstetrical care, but such supervision of the patient before and after delivery by trained nurses and social workers as will make it possible for her to realize the importance of following closely the various regulations laid down for her guidance. In other words, efficient prenatal care must be regarded in great part as a campaign of education for physician and patient, in which both must be taught to realize that ideal obstetrics implies not merely intelligent care at the time of labor, but that it has a much wider scope and should begin as soon as the woman realizes that she is pregnant and continue until she is discharged in ideal physical condition and suckling a normal child."

Recognizing that the social characteristics of most hospital patients could impede the attainment of this ideal, Williams emphasized the need for education by prenatal workers. Only by this means, he said, can the patients "be induced to make the necessary visits to the dispensary before and after delivery, and consequently I have become convinced that efficient prenatal and postnatal care cannot be carried out by physicians alone, and is feasible only when the requisite number of trained nurses and social workers are available."[136]

What this ideal implied was a program carried on within an organization with a staff of trained professionals. This situation could most easily be developed in a health department or hospital clinic, or in a facility operated by a voluntary agency. It was more difficult to do so in the offices of private practitioners. By the early 1920s, maternal and child health activities were accepted preventive functions, even though the implementation of the concept left much to be desired. In 1923, a survey of health department practices in the 100 largest American cities revealed that prenatal clinics were conducted in 73. These clinics were maintained by health departments in 31 cities, by voluntary agencies in 32 cities, and in 10 cities they were supported jointly by governmental and voluntary resources. This was an advance over the situation in 1920 when out of 83 cities with a population of 100,000 or more, almost 50 lacked a prenatal clinic, either public or private. In some of these communities, visiting nurses provided care to pregnant women at home. Throughout this decade the pattern of prenatal care began to take hold and more facilities became available. In Chicago, in 1926, the Health Department maintained 6 clinics, the Infant Welfare Society, a private organization, had 10, and clinics were available in 26 hospitals. However, relatively few women used these services. In very few communities were the clinics attended by as many as 10 percent of the pregnant women. Many were attended by midwives at home. By 1947, nearly 80 percent of the babies born in the United States were delivered in hospitals, and a large proportion of expectant mothers were seeking prenatal care by the third month of pregnancy.[137]

From the efforts at disease prevention and control discussed above it is evident that two basic modes of action were developed and applied in several ways for preventive purposes during the present century. One is modification of the human organism, the other alteration of the human environment. The former includes such measures as specific immunization, chemoprophylaxis, or therapeutic intervention for secondary prevention. Under the latter come such measures as water purification, pasteurization, reduction of air pollution and fortification of food. Given the existence of accurate knowledge concerning disease etiology and pathogenesis, and the availability of effective techniques and organization for application, preventive action is most likely to produce results when it is least subject to socio-economic and cultural constraints or interference. Furthermore, the effectiveness of such action is likely to be enhanced even further when the biological factors in the disease are favorable. Diphtheria is a case in point.

By 1900, diphtheria could be diagnosed by precise bacteriological methods, the sick person could be treated with antitoxin, and carriers could be detected thus making possible effective control. The next important development, direct prevention of the disease, was achieved by active mass immunization, a method developed from earlier knowledge on the use of diphtheria antitoxin as a passive immunizing agent. In 1902, S.K. Dzierzgowsky showed that immunization in a human being could be achieved by increasing doses of diluted toxin. The use of toxin neutralized by antitoxin was then suggested by Theobald Smith in 1909.[138] In 1913, E. von Behring substituted such a mixture for the diluted toxin and demonstrated that it induced immunity safely in animals and man.[139] At the same time it was necessary to know the natural history of diphtheria within the community. How many children of different ages had already acquired immunity, how many were carriers, and which children were highly susceptible? A simple test for immunity by injecting minute amounts of toxin into the skin, developed by Bela Schick in 1913, made it possible to define more accurately the need for active immunization, as well as the results obtained thereby.[140]

Finally, in 1923, G. Ramon showed that toxin treated with formalin (anatoxin, now known as toxoid) had advantages as an immunizing agent over the earlier toxin-antitoxin mixture. Later, alum-precipitated toxoid was found of still greater antigenic potency.

Knowledge and techniques thus became available for a full-scale mass attack on diphtheria, which was first undertaken by William H. Park and Abraham Zingher in New York City. In 1915 Park had immunized several thousand children with toxin-antitoxin and by 1918 it was evident after testing that they had retained their immunity. In 1920, active immunization of school children began, and by 1928 some 500,000 had been immunized.[141] This figure though large represented less than 50 percent of the school child population. Attention was then concentrated on preschool children, and in 1940 it was estimated that no less than 60 percent of this group were protected. By this date, the disease had been virtually eliminated as a cause of death, with a mortality rate of 1.1 per 100,000, as contrasted with a rate of 785 per 100,000 in 1894. With the adoption of immunization in New York and other large cities such as Toronto, and then progressively in other countries, proof of its efficacy became increasingly evident. For many years it was accepted practice to begin diphtheria immunization at about the sixth month. Beginning in the 1940s, however, there has been a trend toward immunizing at progressively earlier ages. This development derived from the finding of the adjuvant effects of combining antigens, for example, diphtheria toxoid with pertussis vaccine, and the fact that a high percentage of susceptible infants responded well to primary immunization against diphtheria when the initial injection is given as early as the second or third month of life.[142]

That the drop in diphtheria morbidity and mortality is not wholly due to preventive immunization appears to be indicated by the fact that this decline set in actually in the 19th century before diphtheria antitoxin began to be used generally, and continued progressively even before preventive immunization became widespread. The death rate among children up to ten years of age in New York City was 785 per 100,000 in 1894, declining to less than 300 in 1900; and in 1920, when active immunization of school children began, it fell below 100. This experience occurred as well in Massachusetts between 1900 and 1940, nor was it limited to these areas. This decline is related not only to the use of antitoxin and passive immunization of contacts, but very likely to a greater extent to the fact that certain communicable diseases, among them diphtheria, occur in waves with intervening periods during which the disease is either absent or at least significantly rarer. Consequently, arguments have been raised against the effectiveness of therapeutic or preventive measures instituted during the waning of an epidemic wave. The German physician Ottomar Rosenbach recognized the cyclical behavior and used it as an argument against claims made for the value of diphtheria antitoxin.[143] Nevertheless, whatever the relative weight of the factors that have brought about a massive decline in cases of diphtheria, it is certain that from a statistical point of view the experience of diphtheria in large urban communities where the disease was concentrated has been significantly better after the introduction of immunization than might have been expected from the trend of either morbidity and mortality in the preimmunization period. Certainly, the downward course of diphtheria morbidity and mortality has at least been accelerated by preventive immunization.[144]

Nevertheless, the disease has not disappeared. In 1959 there were 868 cases in the United States and in 1960 there were 873, most of them concentrated in the southern and southwestern sections of the country among Negro and Latin American groups.[145] In all sections of the country outbreaks occur largely among unimmunized children in such groups characterized by poverty and a low standard of living. These findings call attention to several other aspects of prevention and the use of preventive services.

When diphtheria immunization was introduced, official and voluntary health agencies pushed this program in various ways. Action was taken to involve school children, their parents and teachers, physicians and the general public. In Syracuse during 1923-1928, for example, school children receiving immunizations had their names entered on an honor roll, and received stars for each preschool child brought in by a school child. This aroused classroom competition and helped to publicize the campaign.[146] During the same period, health departments began to develop active programs of immunizations among infants, and made this activity a component of communicable disease control. Immunization was practised within the framework of the child health conference, a form which had developed for the improvement of child health. However, only a relatively small percentage of infants and children could be reached through clinics or such institutions as schools. Slowly, immunization became a part of the armamentarium of the physician who attended pregnant women and the infants to whom they gave birth. As Borden S. Veeder put the matter in 1926, "In private practice the prevention of diphtheria by active immunization is a procedure squarely up to the physician. The means are available and one might almost say that the medical profession as a whole can be judged of its attitude toward preventive medicine by the use it makes of active immunization."[147] In short, patterns of behavior and institutional forms were developing through which immunization could be utilized. These behavioral patterns and the institutions to which they related taught parents to expect that their children need not become ill or die. Furthermore, as new immunizations were developed against tetanus, pertussis, polio, measles and rubella, they have to a greater or lesser extent been incorporated into this arrangement in which pediatricians were most prominent.

But as Charles L. Dana, of the New York Academy of Medicine, observed in 1929, "The usual attitude of the general practitioner toward preventive medicine is of course commendatory but not enthusiastic."[148] On the whole physicians in private practice tended to place little emphasis on prevention, even in the matter of such procedures as smallpox vaccination and diphtheria immunization.[149] Nevertheless, as one generation replaced an earlier one and medical education changed, immunization procedures were accepted and used although inadequacies remained.

As with tuberculosis, diphtheria has retreated to socially peripheral ethnic and racial groups that have not shared in the evolution and utilization of the cultural forms concerned with immunization and other preventive measures for the protection of infants and children. Behavior in relation to health problems in terms of perceiving and coping with them is to a very large extent culturally conditioned and socially learned.[150] Basically, the health status and experience of a given population is a function of its way of life, involving both the social and physical environment. Change to improve health conditions can be brought about in several ways. Change will be accepted more readily if it is introduced as part of a familiar pattern of behavior which is perceived as non-threatening. An example is the use of iodine in table salt to prevent goiter. Similarly, purification of water and sanitation of milk were extremely important in altering the health of Americans young and old, and while these measures aroused some opposition, it was not strong enough to prevent their acceptance. In 1890, only 1.5 percent of the urban population in the United States was supplied with filtered water. By 1914, the proportion was 40 percent, and has continued to rise since then. Chlorination of water supplies did not begin until 1908 and the first national standard for drinking water was issued by the Public Health Service in 1914.[151] Pasteurization of milk has already been discussed in connection with bovine tuberculosis, but some additional effects can be noted here. One is the dramatic decline in typhoid fever, which began in the later 19th century with the introduction of proper sewerage and even more of protected water supplies. Later, further improvements in sanitary engineering, specifically protection of water through purification and of milk through pasteurization, as well as fly control, detection of well carriers, microbiological diagnosis and isolation of patients continued and intensified the earlier trend. Vaccination against typhoid was significant in specific groups, such as military units. By the end of the second decade of this century, the results were evident. In 1900 a group of 20 large cities had typhoid death rates ranging from 13 to 144 per 100,000. By 1920 the rates had been reduced to a range of from 1.1 to 7.4 per 100,000. By 1947 the death rate for the United States was 0.2 per 100,000 for both typhoid and paratyphoid fevers. Children also benefited greatly from the measures described above. From 1915 through 1918 the infant death rate was about 100 per 1000 live births; by 1946 it had dropped to 33.8. The decline has continued since then but at a slower rate. Indeed, this aspect of prevention was succinctly summed up by C.-E.A. Winslow in 1928 when he said, "Typhoid fever has been controlled chiefly by the purification of water supplies, the pasteurization of milk, and the use of vaccine; diphtheria, by the use of antitoxin, and more recently by toxin-antitoxin immunization. . . diarrhea by pasteurization of milk and breast feeding of infants."[152]

Winslow omitted one factor, however, which was particularly important for the efforts to reduce infant morbidity and mortality. Activities concerned with infant health and welfare were aimed to a very large extent at mothers and children in immigrant groups living under poor environmental conditions. The campaign to improve child health must be seen in part as an element in the Americanization movement which had its beginnings at the end of the last century, reached its peak during the First World War, and ebbed away during the 1920s.[153] This movement had several facets, of which one was to combat the exploitation and degradation to which the immigrants weresubjected and "to promote their assimilation, education and advancement."[154] Recognition of the need for social integration of the newer immigration with the older, native America found prominent expression in the establishment of social settlements in the poorest sections of Chicago, New York and other cities.[155] To achieve their aim, the settlement workers turned to the practical problems affecting the immigrant poor, including those concerned with health. It was no accident that the New York Milk Committee, established in 1907 by the Association for Improving the Condition of the Poor, to reduce infant mortality by improving the milk supply, set up infant milk depots in such neighborhoods. Nor was it an accident that in 1911 Wilbur C. Phillips, previously secretary to the Milk Committee, set up his demonstration center for maternal and child care in a Polish district of Milwaukee. This facility was intended as a "centre of influence for child life" where babies could receive medical examinations, where mothers could be taught how to keep their babies well, and from which would "radiate the influences of education and social betterment."[156]

In short, the maternal and infant welfare conferences, the milk stations, the lessons in infant feeding, the school examinations, the campaigns for smallpox vaccination, diphtheria immunization, the use of orange juice and cod liver oil to eliminate scurvy and rickets were intended to reduce infant deaths and improve child health. But these activities also served to assimilate the mother and through her the family to an American way of life. To a greater or lesser degree assimilation occurred and cultural change was accepted. Whatever else the Americanization movement achieved, it helped to advance well-being through cultural assimilation.

This is precisely what did not happen to groups such as Indians, Latin Americans and Blacks who remained peripheral to the mainstream of American culture. A neat demonstration of this phenomenon has been presented by Walsh McDermott and his co-workers on the basis of their Many Farms project over a five year period from 1955 to 1960.[157] Despite the availability of good medical care, infant morbidity and mortality, due chiefly to diarrhea and pheumonia were not reduced. Essentially these conditions are the consequence of poor sanitary conditions as well as improper and inadequate nutrition, precisely the same factors responsible for high infant mortality among the urban poor earlier in the century. As long as such a population group maintains a culture pattern in which pathogenic factors persist, it would be difficult to alter the occurrence of disease. Preventive measures will be effective only insofar as they can be introduced and implemented within a changed way of life.

Such a change need not be a matter of individual or group volition. A good example is the disappearance of pellagra in the United States. Beginning around 1907, there was an increase in the incidence as well as in the recognition of the disease in the United States, especially in the South.[158] By the end of 1909, it was reported from 26 states. In 1916, pellagra ranked second among the causes of death in South Carolina. Joseph Goldberger was assigned by the Public Health Service in 1914 to study the problem, and by the following year he demonstrated that the disease was due to some inadequacy in the diet of pellagra sufferers.[159] When the diet was improved by the addition of milk and fresh meat, the disease disappeared, breaking out again when the faulty diet was restored. But what was the exact element in the diet which when absent caused pellagra? By 1920 Goldberger suggested that a vitamin factor (pellagra preventive) might be involved. Subsequently, Goldberger demonstrated that the anti-beriberi substance, the B factor, was also a specific for pellagra, and in 1926 he reported that the B factor consisted of two components, the one effective against beriberi, the other against pellagra.

How pellagra could be prevented or cured was thus largely known by the late 1920s, but the disease was not overcome until two decades later. The reason lay not in a lack of knowledge, although not all problems had been solved, but rather in the economic and social factors that affected the dietary of the cotton raising South. Goldberger was fully aware of this aspect of the problem, and together with Edgar Sydenstricker carried out a series of classic studies in the social epidemiology of pellagra. Some were carried out in cotton mill villages, others among tenant farmers.[160] An unmistakeable inverse correlation between family income and pellagra incidence was demonstrated. However, income was not the only factor involved. Sources of food supply and dietary habits played important roles as well. When families in mill villages were restricted to the mill store or commissary during the late winter or spring because of the absence of other sources of supply, and given the restricted food pattern of the poorer class in the South, pellagra was almost inevitable. Furthermore, the conomic condition of the rural popultion was tied to the tenant system and single-crop agricultural production, chiefly cotton. As a result of the speculative nature of agricultural financing in this situation, tenant income tended to fluctuate rapidly from one season to the next. According to Rupert B. Vance, writing in 1929, "cotton growing is a more or less haphazard game of see-saw between production on one hand and demand as represented by prices on the other."[161] Tenant farmers mortgaged their prospective crops and hoped for high prices, but if the crop failed or prices fell, income was non-existent and the diet extremely restricted. Unfavorable cotton years were followed by an increased incidence of pellagra. Goldberger could recommend the keeping of cows and chicken, and the planting of gardens, but he could not change the economics of the situation.

This change was achieved by the depression of the thirties and the Second World War. The collapse of the cotton market led the federal government to institute a policy of reducing cotton acreage and destroying cotton crops in the fields. Concomitantly, the Agricultural Extension Service urged farmers to grow food crops for home use.[162] The Farm Security Administration provided needy tenant farmers with cookstoves where there had been only a hearth, mules and wagons, as well as pressure cookers so that surplus food could be canned. It was in essence a program of mass adult education.[163] But this was only a beginning. Although there was some decline in the number of reported cases and deaths following the institution of these programs, pellagra did not disappear. Not until the Second World War was it finally conquered. The war brought a greater increase in employment, and together with mobilization of the armed forces provided practically everyone with an adequate income as well as the possibility of securing a better diet, particularly in high protein food. The demise of endemic pellagra was further hastened by the food enrichment program, particularly the enrichment of bread during the war, which has already been discussed.[164] One more factor must be added. Throughout this period and particularly since the war, the South has become increasingly urbanized, industrialized, and agriculture has become diversified. With better transportation facilities the South has moved into the mainstream of American culture affecting standards of living.[165]

The implications of pellagra prevention are quite clear. Food is a necessity for the maintenance of life, but it is also inextricably linked with culturally conditioned behavior and with forms of economic organization. As a result various groups in the United States, particularly those with low incomes continue to suffer from malnutrition. Nutrition research and education remain as necessary as ever, but it is evident that improvement of nutrition basically involves economic, social and political questions. When action is taken along these lines on the basis of valid knowledge, malnutrition and its consequences can be prevented.

Within the limits of this analysis, it is manifestly impossible to discuss many specific health problems in detail. It is clear, however, that during the 40 years from 1900 to the outbreak of the Second World War disease prevention and health promotion developed along specific lines in the United States. Basically, these activities were divided into community and individual services. The former included the collection and analysis of vital statistics; the control of communicable diseases, including tuberculosis, syphilis and gonorrhea; maternity, infant and child hygiene; school health supervision; sanitation; food and milk control; laboratory services required for the performance of the aforementioned activities; public health nursing, and public health education. The individual services included immunization and periodic health examination. Obviously this classification used by Lee and Jones in 1933 is not entirely satisfactory, as they acknowledged.[166] The bulk of these services were provided by local and state health departments with support and cooperation from the federal government, chiefly through the Public Health Service, and from voluntary health agencies, usually concerned with specific problems or population groups. The role of the medical and dental professions was more limited, acting through professional organizations or in private practice. Thus, immunizations could be administered in private practice, by general physicians or pediatricians, or in clinics run by official or voluntary agencies. Similarly periodic check-ups of pregnant women, infants and children could be provided privately as well as through community agencies. Clinical practitioners could supervise patients with tuberculosis or venereal diseases, but the cases had to be reported and checks were made by the official health agency to make sure that transmission did not occur because of poor personal hygiene. This was also the case with the acute communicable diseases such as diphtheria, scarlet fever, typhoid or pneumonia.

Taken as a whole the goals of community health action were clearly envisaged within an accepted program, and institutional forms were available to encompass the diversity of knowledge and professional identity which emerged with the expansion of public health and preventive medicine in the earlier decades of this century. Essentially, this involved the control of bacterial pollution in the environment, the prevention of communicable diseases, parasitic infestations, and the morbid conditions produced by defective nutrition, and the achievement of these aims through an official agency, complemented in various ways by voluntary health agencies and clinical practitioners. Although the participants in these three sectors did not always see eye to eye, and conflicts sometimes occurred, the system worked on the whole.[167] Basically, this pattern remained changed until after the Second World War. Some jurisdictions included dental services for children, and particularly on the state level increasing attention was given to the problem of occupational health.[168]

Recognition that there were not enough local health agencies staffed by competent, trained personnel appeared at the end of the 19th century and spread in subsequent decades. Hermann Biggs, in 1897, called attention to the need to train physicians for careers in public health, and advocated the establishment of a school for this purpose. In 1908, Norman E. Ditman of New York urged the creation of a "school of preventive medicine" to train future health officers. The following year, Irving Fisher, the Yale economist, emphasized the need to secure special training "for what is really a new profession, that of public health officer." He proposed that "the curricula of medical schools should be rearranged with greater emphasis on prevention and on the training of health officers." Fisher also called attention to a committee of the American Medical Association, of which he was a member, which had been appointed to study and improve medical schools. In 1913, a sub-committee of this group, comprising Charles V. Chapin, John S. Fulton, Milton J. Rosenau, Victor C. Vaughan, and Fisher, issued a report calling for institutes of public health, financed and equipped to offer instruction and to carry on research. This group also urged the organized teaching of preventive medicine to medical students, and the development of courses for health officers and allied professional groups.[169] As early as 1908, Chapin had expressed the hope that every health officer would be trained for his work. This view was reinforced by a survey of state public health work which he carried out during 1914 and the early part of 1915 at the request of the council on Health and Public Instruction of the American Medical Association. The report of this survey appeared in 1916, emphasizing among numerous findings the need for qualified men.[170]

This trend was strengthened by the experience and observations of the Rockefeller Sanitary Commission established in 1909 to combat the ravages of hookworm and its devastating economic, social and cultural consequences in the rural South. From a survey conducted in 1910 by Wickliffe Rose, director of the Commission, it became clear that an effective county health service administered by a capable health officer was essential if the program for prevention and control of hookworm infestation was to succeed. This need and the efforts to meet it represent a constant theme in the development of educational programs and institutions intended to prepare trained personnel to provide preventive services. In 1914, Louis I. Dublin, statistician at the Metropolitan Life Insurance Company and a leader in public health, developed a plan for county health units administered by full-time health officers "trained in the science of sanitation and public health."[171] Similar ideas were expressed by John A. Ferrell, director of the International Health Board of the Rockefeller Foundation.[172]

Meanwhile, the Rockefeller Foundation at the urging of Wickliffe Rose set in motion a study by Abraham Flexner which led to the establishment in June, 1916, of the School of Hygiene and Public Health at the Johns Hopkins University with William H. Welch as director. Rose and Welch proposed that the School educate and train the various kinds of specialists and experts required in public health. These included full-time health officers for federal, state and local service, statisticians, epidemiologists, sanitary engineers, chemists, bacteriologists, public health nurses and sanitary inspectors. Furthermore, it was intended to overcome

"first, the lack of a sufficiently broad and sound basis of scientific knowledge for the systematic promotion of public and personal hygiene; second, the lack of a well-defined career as an attraction to able men whose interest is in this field rather in the practice of medicine; third, the lack of due emphasis, in the training of practitioners of medicine, upon the importance of hygiene and of the practitioner's role as an apostle of hygiene no less than therapy."[173]

The third point touches on a very important aspect of disease prevention, namely, the role of the clinical practitioner in the performance of this function and his preparation for it, a subject of increasing interest and significance at present. To judge by the available evidence, preventive medicine has never been a popular subject among medical students or medical practitioners. In 1953, J.M. Mackintosh, professor of public health at the University of London observed,

"Everyone says that prevention is better than cure, and hardly anyone acts as if he believes it. . . . Palliatives nearly always take precedence over prevention, and our health services today are too heavily loaded with salvage. Treatment—the attempt to heal the sick—is more tangible, more exciting and more immediately rewarding, than prevention."[174]

Seven years earlier, in 1946, Perrin H. Long, professor of preventive medicine at the Johns Hopkins Medical School, reported that a large number of medical students wanted "instruction in public health (preventive medicine) . . . deemphasized."[175] A related point was made in 1942 by George Baehr, E.H.L. Corwin and James A. Miller when they said,

"Because of the advances of medical knowledge, the medical school curriculum has become so crowded that the social importance of preventive medicine and public health is seldom emphasized. This creates a blind spot which often persists throughout professional life and results at times in misunderstandings between the practicing physicians and the constituted health authorities of the community."[176]

Nor is the situation much better at present, to judge by the comments of Milton Terris, who with grim humor suggests that perhaps medical schools should be administratively responsible to schools of public health in which case the former might be encouraged to educate physicians interested in preventive medicine and its application to benefit the health of the public.[177]

This situation with respect to preventive medicine and public health is due to economic, social and cultural factors which have determined the socio-economic philosophy of most members of the medical profession and the social logic within which they perceive behavior and values related to health action. These attitudes and views are of long standing. In their studies of Middletown from 1925 to 1935 the Lynds commented in 1937 that

> "the attitude of the majority of Middletown's doctors regarding private practice and public health facilities remains substantially that described in 1925. All proposals to develop clinical facilities of whatever type in Middletown still operate within the straitjacket of insistence by the majority of the local medical profession that nothing shall be done to make Middletown healthier that jeopardizes the position of the doctors."[178]

Another factor is the matter of status relations. Medical practitioners have generally held in low esteem those physicians who did not engage in private practice and ventured into other fields of health activity. As Carey P. McCord describes this attitude, a physician in the opinion of many of his professional brethren

> "may be in only four places—at the bedside, in the consultation room, in the hospital, at the academy of medicine. With a fair degree of tolerance these physicians accept the insurance doctor, the ship's physician, the medical public health officer, the medical teacher and the military surgeon, but rarely are they taken into the profession's bosom. Their enterprises are regarded as rather unfortunate happenings, though not entirely deplorable."[179]

To a certain extent this attitude reflects the disdain present in our society for anyone who does not elect to follow the individualistic, competitive pattern of the culture. The findings reported in 1959 by Coker *et al.* on public health as seen through the eyes of medical students tend to support this point. Furthermore, the clinical practitioner is still basically oriented to the individual patient, since most of those practising today were trained a generation or so ago. Whether medical students trained in more recent years are different remains to be seen.

In any event during the early years of the century, "private practitioners of medicine" were "most useful in the diagnosis and treatment of disease and in the advising of individuals and families regarding disease prevention and health promotion," noted Lewellys F. Barker. However, he went on to observe that though

> "it is only relatively recently that the public-health services have entered the fields of diagnostic and curative medicine (left formerly entirely to private practice) . . . experience with public medical and nursing services for maternal and child welfare; for the health of school children; for the

early recognition and proper treatment of certain infectious diseases ... would indicate that public-health workers will from now on become even more active in diagnostic and curative domains."[180]

The point made by Barker in a prophetic mood touches on the accommodation between medical and public health practitioners in the area of disease prevention, a situation which was unstable but which could be maintained as long as no major disturbing factors intruded. This accommodation was possible because the problems with which public health practitioners were concerned did not impinge on private practice, or affected specific groups of the population, most of which were poor and unable to afford private care, or because the official health agency provided services useful to the private practitioner. To the extent to which public health separated its province of action (vital statistics, environmental sanitation, health education, public health nursing etc.) by maintaining relatively distinct boundaries, this situation could be maintained. Even diagnosis and treatment of venereal diseases and tuberculosis, or the provision of prenatal and infant care, could be accepted as long as these services did not affect the sphere which the private practitioner considered his own.

Under these conditions, public health practitioners could carry on programs, and schools of public health could teach them their place in the health arena, and provide them with the knowledge to carry out their tasks. For the overwhelming majority of medical students and their teachers, intent on the diagnosis and treatment of disease, the concept of prevention and its implementation through community action had little attraction or apparent relevance, since it did not fit into the professional structure of medical practice.[181] During this very period, the decades preceding the Second World War, however, changes were taking shape which would disrupt this situation, and confront the United States with new problems requiring new solutions, problems that would require a rethinking of preventive medicine and public health.

ILLUSTRATIONS

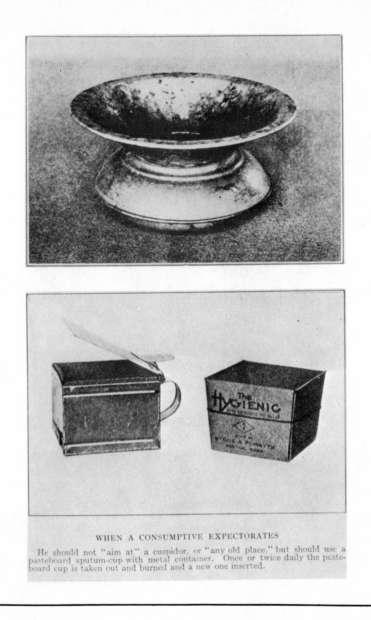

WHEN A CONSUMPTIVE EXPECTORATES

He should not "aim at" a cuspidor, or "any old place," but should use a pasteboard sputum-cup with metal container. Once or twice daily the pasteboard cup is taken out and burned and a new one inserted.

1 Personal hygiene was considered an important facet of tuberculosis control, and special attention was given to expectoration of sputum and to its sanitary disposal. FROM G.L. HOWE: *How to Prevent Sickness*, NEW YORK, 1918.

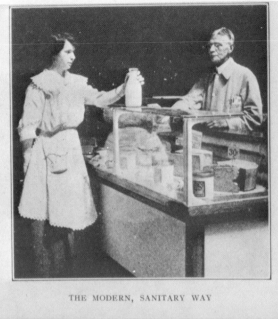

THE MODERN, SANITARY WAY

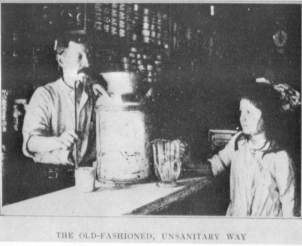

THE OLD-FASHIONED, UNSANITARY WAY

2 Food sanitation was a major approach to the prevention of communicable disease during the early decades of the 20th century. Dispensing pasteurized milk in bottles or other closed containers rather than from open cans was an important step toward this objective. FROM HOWE, 1918.

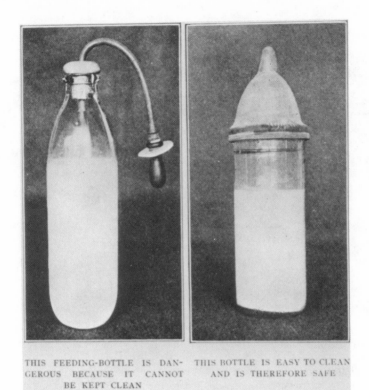

THIS FEEDING-BOTTLE IS DAN-
GEROUS BECAUSE IT CANNOT
BE KEPT CLEAN

THIS BOTTLE IS EASY TO CLEAN
AND IS THEREFORE SAFE

3 Similarly attention was given to the sanitation of infant feeding utensils in order to prevent diarrhea. FROM HOWE, 1918.

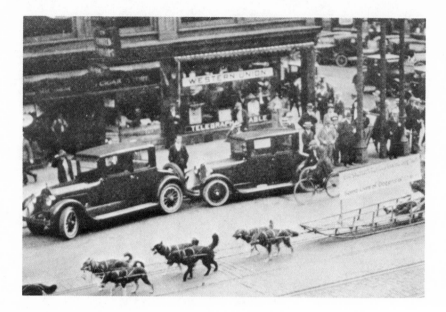

The antidiphtheria campaign was publicized by Shannon's dog team.

4   Recognition of the need to inform and to involve various elements of the community in preventive programs led to the development of health education, employing publicity, advertising and various other methods during the 1920s and successive decades. An example is this action to publicize diphtheria immunization using the occasion of a diphtheria epidemic in Nome, Alaska in the 1920s when antitoxin was brought to the city by dog-sled. The driver and his dog team were brought to Syracuse where they paraded the streets of the city during the noon hour to stress the importance of diphtheria immunization. FROM LOUISE F. BACHE: *Health Education in an American City. . .* , NEW YORK, 1934.

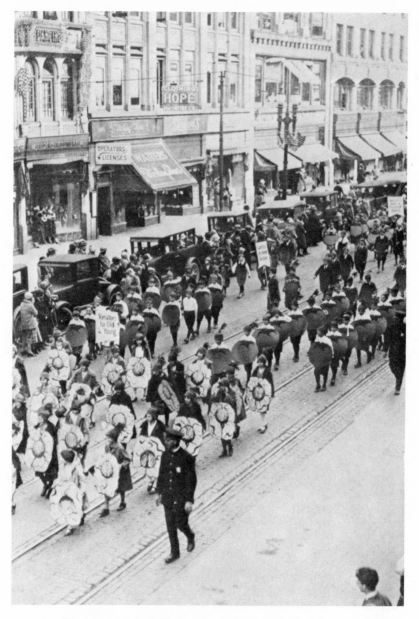

The vegetable battalion in the annual health parade.

5 Advertising the importance of good nutrition in the City of Syracuse, an example of health education in the 1920s. FROM BACHE, 1934.

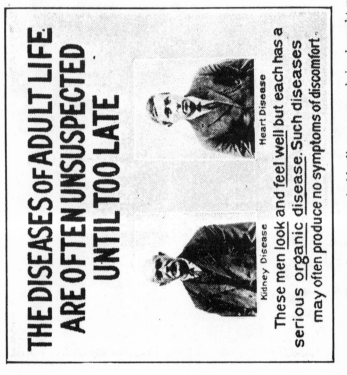

THE DISEASES OF ADULT LIFE ARE OFTEN UNSUSPECTED UNTIL TOO LATE

Kidney Disease

Heart Disease

These men look and feel well but each has a serious organic disease. Such diseases may often produce no symptoms of discomfort.

6 At the same time that communicable diseases were being brought under control through preventive measures, attention began to be given to important non-communicable diseases and to the necessity for their early detection. This point was increasingly stressed during the second and third decades of the century. FROM HOWE, 1918.

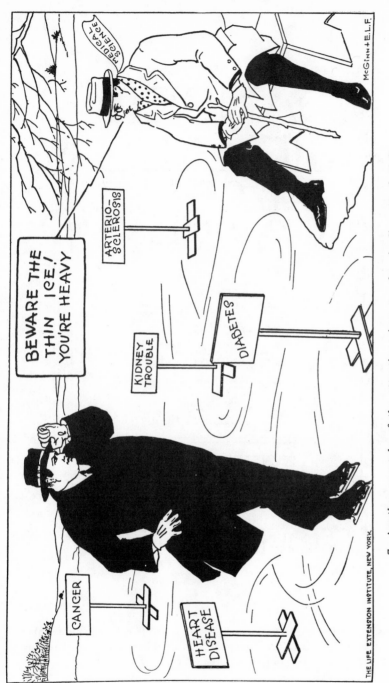

7 Another example of the attention given to chronic diseases of adults. FROM *How To Live. A Monthly Journal of Health and Hygiene*, NOVEMBER, 1930.

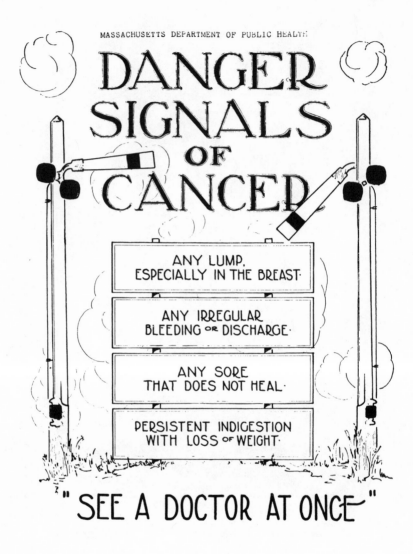

DANGER SIGNALS OF CANCER

ANY LUMP, ESPECIALLY IN THE BREAST·

ANY IRREGULAR BLEEDING OR DISCHARGE·

ANY SORE THAT DOES NOT HEAL·

PERSISTENT INDIGESTION WITH LOSS OF WEIGHT·

"SEE A DOCTOR AT ONCE"

8 An aspect of the increasing attention given to chronic, non-communicable diseases was action to inform the public, as in this circular issued by the Massachusetts Department of Health, circa 1928.

The Menace of Middle Age

Medical Society of the County of
New York
DeWitt Stetten, M. D., President
Medical Society of the County of
Kings
Thomas M. Brennan, M. D.,
President
Bronx County Medical Society
Harry Aranow, M. D., President
Medical Society of the County of
Queens
William J. Lavelle, M. D., President
Richmond County Medical Society
George Walrath, M. D., President

can be met by the practice of Health Examinations

CONTRARY to the experience in other civilized countries where the death rate has improved at every age period in the past decade, the death rate at middle life and later is increasing in the United States.

Loss in Expectation of Life at Certain Ages

Age	1921	1927	Loss
37	32.86	31.47	1.39 years
47	28.90	27.51	1.39 "
57	17.72	16.57	1.15 "
67	11.50	10.60	.90 "

The loss indicated by these figures may seem numerically small, but occurring in the most vital years and, contrasted with the gains in other countries, it is serious and a warning of the need for action.

This increasing death rate is caused by a class of diseases that usually pass unrecognized by the sufferer. The magnitude of the problem, and the public menace of these diseases is shown in the latest available statistics for the United States Registration Area, where there were reported in

1926, 1,285,927 deaths. Four or five outstanding preventable diseases contributed nearly one - half of this mortality.

The foremost medical men of our time agree that the practice of periodic health examinations could detect and control these diseases in their incipient stages. Even when these diseases are discovered too late for complete cure, it is possible for scientific control to modify their course.

Diseases not now on the increase, such as tuberculosis, are still too prevalent. The periodic health examination is a fundamental measure in the great warfare against all disease, and is not limited to the chronic maladies which constitute an outstanding menace.

Apart from the discovery of many of the causes of these maladies, and their cure or mitigation, the periodic health examination and the medical and hygienic instructions based upon them will help to build up vitality and make stronger men, women and children.

HAVE A HEALTH EXAMINATION
Not in Fear of Disease, But for the Love of Health

Greater New York Committee on Health Examination
──────────New York County Committee──────────

A. J. Rongy, M. D., *Chairman*   S. Dana Hubbard, M. D.   Orrin S. Wightman, M. D.
Iago Galdston, M. D., *Secretary*   Frederic W. Bancroft, M. D.   Linsly R. Williams, M. D.
Eugene L. Fisk, M. D.

Chairman Kings County Committee   Chairman Bronx County Committee
Alec N. Thomson, M. D.   Louis A. Friedman, M. D.

Chairman Queens County Committee   Chairman Richmond County Committee
William J. Lavelle, M. D.   A. E. Bernstein, M. D.

Contributed by Milbank Memorial Fund, New York Tuberculosis & Health Association, Metropolitan Life Insurance Company, Brooklyn Tuberculosis & Health Association, Life Extension Institute, and Queensboro Tuberculosis & Health Association.

9   The concept of the periodic health examination as a preventive measure came into prominence in the 1920s and was pushed by life insurance companies, medical societies, health departments, voluntary health agencies, and other groups interested in prevention of disease. This statement was issued by the New York County Medical Society in the late 1920s.

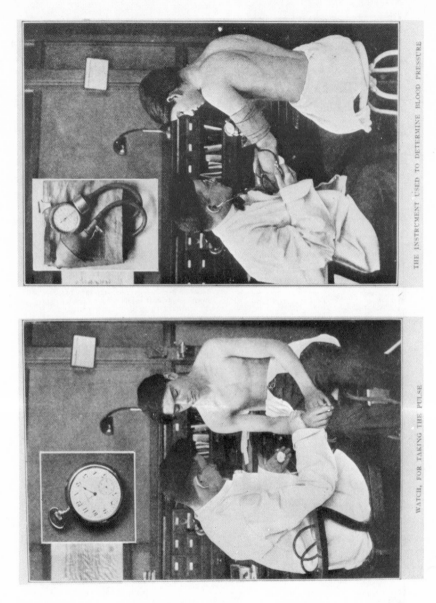

10   The periodic health examination as conceived and practised during the period 1910-1940 was simple, comprising essentially a history, physical examination, some laboratory tests (urinalysis, blood examination) and

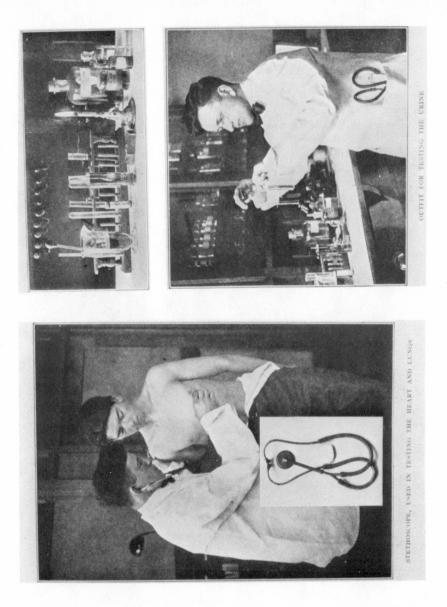

possibly fluoroscopy or chest plate. The four illustrations shown here are from a book intended for a non-professional audience and present some steps in the health examination. FROM HOWE, 1918.

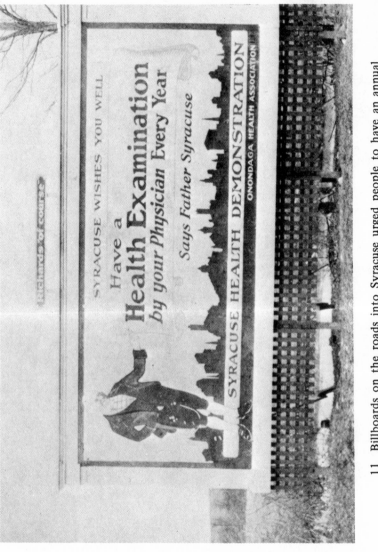

11 Billboards on the roads into Syracuse urged people to have an annual health examination. FROM BACHE, 1934.

What Periodic Health Examinations Reveal

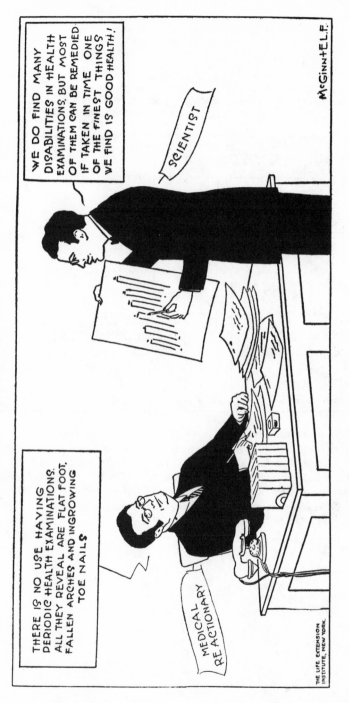

12 Numerous physicians felt that periodic health examinations were not worth the time expended on them since no serious pathological conditions were discovered. This cartoon from a publication issued by the Life Extension Institute in 1931 presents arguments for and against such examinations. FROM *How To Live. A Monthly Journal of Health and Hygiene,* MARCH, 1931.

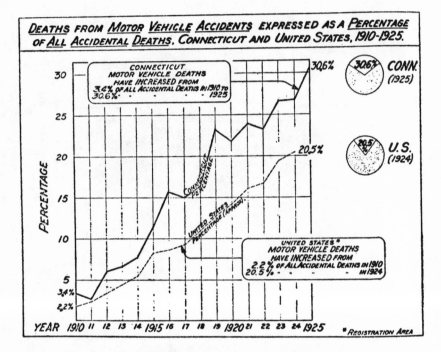

Deaths from Motor Vehicle Accidents expressed as a Percentage of All Accidental Deaths, Connecticut and United States, 1910-1925.

13 Deaths and injuries resulting from motor vehicle accidents are today still a major public health problem even though the problem was recognized over fifty years ago. As indicated by this chart for the period 1910-1925, the rising trend of automotive deaths was already clear by the third decade of this century. FROM R.B. STOECKEL, MOTOR VEHICLE ACCIDENT PREVENTION, *DeLamar Lectures, Johns Hopkins School of Hygiene 1925-1926*, BALTIMORE, 1927.

Mr. Auto Fiend Runs Neck and Neck with Influenza and Easily Beats
Typhoid Fever in the Marathon of Death

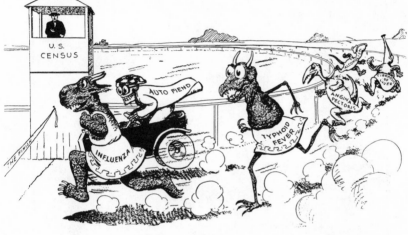

14 By the end of the 1920s it was already evident that mortality from communicable diseases was declining in significance relative the chronic or non-communicable conditions, among them motor vehicle accidents. FROM *How To Live. A Monthly Journal of Health and Hygiene*, AUGUST, 1929.

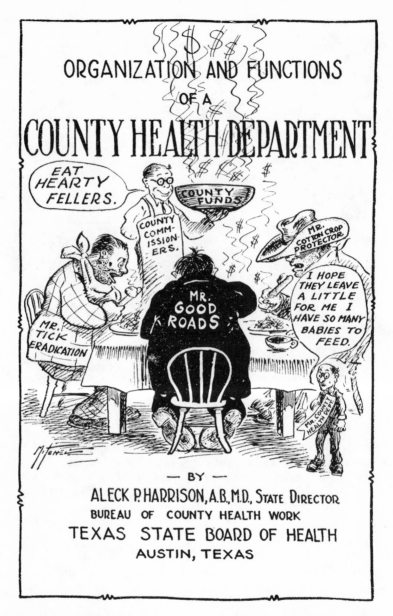

15 Inadequacies in the programs of local health departments have not infrequently been due to financial malnutrition, so that stress on county health units and their functions was frequently presented in terms of adequate appropriations. An example is this cartoon from a pamphlet issued by the Texas State Board of Health, ca. 1920-1925.

Population Change
Chronic Disease
and New Problems

Some 50 years ago it was already apparent that there were strikingly unequal rates of change in various sectors of our society. Some were altering rapidly, while others were lagging by comparison. Even then it was evident that these unequal rates of change in different areas of social life were creating points of tension and zones of social conflict. One of these was that scientific discovery and technologic innovation with respect to health and disease were outstripping the development of organization for their most effective utilization. Advances in medical science led to the use of new diagnostic and curative procedures and instruments. These developments together with the growth of urbanization led to the centralization of medical care in the hospital. Access to medical care was facilitated by this process, but at the same time the cost of medical care increased and complicated its distribution. As a result, a realization emerged that medical service for an industrialized urban society required new forms of financing and organization. Since then, this question has remained a major social and health problem with the important repercussions on preventive medicine and public health.[182]

Paralleling this trend, another significant line of change emerged as a consequence of the very success of disease prevention and control. The introduction of the sulfonamide drugs in the late 1930s and the antibiotics in the mid-1940s accelerated the declining mortality rates for a number of infectious diseases among them puerperal sepsis, scarlet fever, erysipelas, meningococcal meningitis, pneumonia as well as others, such as tuberculosis (discussed above). The introduction of penicillin led to a dramatic drop in the syphilis mortality rate, accelerating a decline that had begun following the intensive campaign against the disease initiated in 1936 by Thomas Parran. Though the disease has not been eliminated and continues to be an important health problem, the sequelae of primary syphilis have largely disappeared or been drastically diminished.[183] Acute rheumatic fever and its sequelae affecting the heart and the kidney have also been removed as significant health problems through chemoprophylaxis. Success has also been achieved with vaccines for poliomyelitis, measles and rubella.

With the decline in morbidity and mortality from communicable respiratory and gastrointestinal diseases, particularly in children and young adults, life expectancy at birth increased. Larger numbers of people live longer and more people survive into older age groups associated with the non-communicable diseases, the so-called degenerative diseases. As a result, among the problems that confront us are such chronic ailments as cancer, cardio-vascular and renal conditions, diabetes mellitus, arthritis, musculoskeletal conditions, and mental changes associated with ageing. Due to better diagnostic facilities

55

and techniques, these conditions are undoubtedly identified more often. Nevertheless, their increasing incidence has been real and is most likely due to the aging of the population. These trends were already evident almost forty years ago.[184] Owing to the impossibility of discussing all chronic diseases in a limited space, only a few conditions will be treated to illustrate some basic aspects of prevention and control.

Consideration of cancer as a preventable disease appears early in the century, even though approached in a simple manner. Woods Hutchinson in 1909 noted that the disease was related to advancing years in that most cases occurred between the ages of forty and sixty. He also observed that most malignant growths in women developed in the uterus and the breasts. For prevention of cancer he recommended avoidance of chronic inflammation and irritation of warts and birthmarks, since these "show a distinctly greater tendency than normal tissue to develop into cancer. Cracks, fissures, chafes and ulcers of all sorts, especially about the lips, tongue, mammary gland, uterus and rectum, should be early and antiseptically dealt with."[185] Once the disease has started the only remedy of any value is surgery.

A somewhat more pessimistic note was struck in 1918 by G.L. Howe, medical director of the Eastman Kodak Company, who stated bluntly that "cancer cannot really be prevented, as it is apt to occur in spite of anything we may do to prevent it."[186] Certain precautions, however, may lessen the chances of cancer, and more probably may increase the probability of cure. These are: an annual physical examination, which cannot be relied on alone, avoidance of unusual or persistent irritation of any part of the body, such as that produced by excessive smoking or a sharp tooth, and prompt attendance to bleeding warts or moles, or tears of the uterine cervix, and medical consultation if there is loss of weight, persistent indigestion, chronic ulcerations in the mouth, or a lump in the breast. Furthermore, a lump in the breast should be removed for microscopical examination, and x-ray examination should also be employed. If cancer is found, surgical removal is the treatment of choice, but x-rays and radium are also mentioned for therapy.

In 1925, Francis Carter Wood, director of the Institute of Cancer Research at Columbia University, urged the need to educate the public if cancer was to be controlled. "Despite all improvements in surgery," he said, "no change has taken place in the recorded death rate." Therefore, the public should be informed to seek medical aid as soon as any suspicious signs and symptoms appear. People "must be taught to consult a physician promptly, and after the age of forty-five, which is the time when cancer becomes a menace, to have yearly examinations, especially if there is a history of cancer in the family." Wood also emphasized the need to educate the physician so that there would be as little delay as possible in making a diagnosis and referring the patient for treatment.[187]

Public health authorities also recognized cancer as a very important health problem. But the question was what to do about it. Eugene R. Kelley, Health Commissioner of Massachusetts, expressed the position of the public health administrator in 1923, when he urged his colleagues to determine "just what their proper niche is in the cancer struggle."[188] Other needs, he said, were better statistical data to establish the dimensions and other characteristics of the problem, more facilities for early diagnosis and stimulation of professionals to use them, and more and better methods to arouse and retain public interest and understanding of the cancer problem. Supporting this position was the view expressed editorially the following year in the *American Journal of Public Health*. According to the writer, the study of cancer had not revealed any general causes as was the case with infectious diseases, so that

> "it is impossible to formulate any program of general measures which offers hope of success in actually preventing the occurrence of cancer. The problem has resolved itself, therefore, quite definitely into one of educating the general population to recognize the early signs of cancer on the one hand, and of providing such clinical facilities as are necessary accurately to diagnose and properly to treat those persons who believe they recognize these early signs and apply for assistance."[189]

The viewpoints expressed by those concerned with cancer must be seen within the setting of developments between 1900 and 1937 when the National Cancer Institute was established. In 1900, the death rate for cancer was about 64 per 100,000 population. The rate climbed steadily early in the century and by 1926 had reached 114. In 1900 cancer was eighth among the leading causes of death, but by 1933 it had reached second place, where it still remained in 1960, with a death rate of 147.4 per 100,000. Whether this was a real or an apparent increase was much debated during the earlier period, but by 1926 Louis I. Dublin concluded that "cancer as a cause of disability and death is increasing" stressing that "there is no longer any room for doubt about that."[190]

Meanwhile, various beginnings to study cancer systematically had been undertaken. The American Medical Association had formed a Committee on Collective Cancer Investigation in 1905. Cancer research at Memorial Hospital in New York City began in 1910, and the Institute of Cancer Research at Columbia University was established in 1911. Some action was also taken by public health authorities. Beginning 1896, the Massachusetts Health Department had collected statistics on cancer and studied its incidence. These investigations were supplemented after 1919 by a diagnostic cancer service to which physicians could refer patients and by a limited health education program.[191] The United States Public Health Service in 1922 sponsored a small laboratory for cancer research headed by Joseph W. Schereschewsky at the Harvard Medical School, and the same year Carl Voegtlin began to investigate cancer at the Hygienic Laboratory in Washington. An analysis of the 1900 to 1920 cancer mortality experience in the Death Registration Area was published in 1925 by Schereschewsky.[192] Cancer control was also a matter of considerable interest to certain medical specialists, principally gynecologists and surgeons, who took steps to establish a voluntary organization "to collect, collate and disseminate the information concerning the symptoms, diagnosis, treatment and prevention of cancer; to investigate the conditions under which cancer is found, and to compile statistics thereto."[193] In 1913, the American Society for the Control of Cancer came into being. As in the case of similar organizations, the Society endeavored to work with professional and lay groups. Since little was known about the biology of cancer, a term covering a variety of conditions, efforts were made to convince physicians and patients (actual or potential) that cancer is curable if discovered and treated in an early stage; to provide accurate information about the disease so as to dispel myths and fears; to encourage health departments to develop programs for cancer control and to urge the participation of state and county medical societies in such activities through cancer committees and personal action.

Thus through the first 40 years of the century, cancer control developed along three lines: education and information, early diagnosis, and research. Clearly knowledge was necessary for effective prevention, preferably primary. But as long as valid knowledge was inadequate, recourse was had to the first two methods which appeared feasible and likely to be beneficial. Moreover, this approach was congruent with a mode of prevention which achieved prominence at the same time, the periodic health examination. The idea of a medical examination at regular intervals of apparently well individuals for the detection of inapparent pathological conditions was first broached by Horace Dobell, an English physician in 1861, but aroused little interest. Around the turn of the century, however, several physicians in Europe and the United States revived the idea.[194] The idea found a congenial environment in the movement, described above, for the protection of health as a way of conserving human resources. One of its chief proponents was a physician, Eugene Lyman Fisk, who as medical director of the Provident Savings Life Association in 1909 organized a free periodic health examination system and an educational service for the company's policy holders.[195] This initial program led in 1913 to the founding of the Life Extension Institute, an enterprise supported by Irving Fisher, Lee K. Frankel and others prominent in the movement for health conservation, with Fisk as medical director. At an annual fee of $20, an individual would receive a health examination and be able to participate in all educational activities of the Institute. In 1914, the Metropolitan Life Insurance Company, also interested in health protection for its policy holders, arranged for the Institute to give them free examinations. The executives of the company were aware of the changing disease picture in the United

States and believed that this measure would benefit their policy holders.[196] This development received additional impetus in 1922 when the House of Delegates of the American Medical Association voted to promote periodic health examinations as a measure for health protection and promotion through state and county medical societies. This step was taken in part at the request of the National Health Council and the American Public Health Association. As is not uncommon under such circumstances in the United States, a crusade for periodic examinations soon followed. This movement was fueled by several different forces. First was the impression derived from recruits examined during the First World War of the defective health status of many Americans. Second was the desire on the part of many voluntary health agencies to propagandize the public for early diagnosis as in cancer. Thirdly, one must remember that the organized medical profession had just come through its first campaign in opposition to the first efforts for compulsory health insurance, but had not yet retreated into a monolithic refusal to accept any public or community effort that appeared to threaten private fee-for-service practice. The periodic examination did not appear to be a threat since it was proposed that the general practitioner stimulate "interest in periodic medical examinations on the part of his own patients so that he may practice preventive medicine, by the use of his own diagnostic skill, in his own private office."[197] In fact, on its face, this proposal would seem to enhance the position of the practitioner in the community.

The campaign that began in 1922 endeavored to have physicians perform examinations, and to have people seek them. Between 1922 and 1929 medical and other periodicals, newspapers and other communications media urged the public to be examined, explained how examinations were performed, and reported on the findings among those examined. In 1925, the A.M.A. issued a handbook, *A Manual of Suggestions for the Conduct of Periodic Examinations of Apparently Healthy Persons*, and the following year E.L. Fisk and J.R. Crawford published *How to Make the Periodic Health Examination*. Essentially, the health examination comprised three parts: history, physical examination including a pelvic examination for women, and a rectal examination for both men and women; and laboratory tests (urinalysis, blood count, serological test for syphilis), chest x-ray or fluoroscopy, and EKG for those over 40, especially men.[198] Blank forms were available from the American Medical Association, and an examination form suitable for infants and children was recommended by the American Child Health Association.

On July 4, 1923, the National Health Council launched a campaign for periodic health examination under the slogan, "Have a Health Examination on Your Birthday." Medical societies, health departments, and voluntary health agencies took action to implement the idea.[199] "It may be correct in theory," Kant entitled one of his essays, implying that the particular concept would not work in practice, and this is indeed an apt summary of the periodic examination campaign. After a few years it was clear that the hopes placed in it would not be realized.

There were a number of reasons why the campaign failed due to factors influencing both the physician and the patient. For most physicians the periodic medical examination simply did not fit into the pattern of practice. Their medical education and training had oriented them to the diagnosis of disease and its treatment, not to prevention, except in a few limited areas such as immunization and avoiding deficiency diseases. Furthermore, as one physician observed, "Private practice has one disadvantage—it is primarily organized to meet emergencies"—examinations "must be planned for in advance—they require the doctor's uninterrupted time."[200] In addition, there was an assumption that the person interested in a health examination usually had a private physician, an assumption that certainly did not apply to the many low-income patients who attended dispensaries or sought private medical care only when absolutely essential. This raises the question of cost, both in time and money, which does not seem to have been considered seriously by the advocates of such examinations. Finally, there was the basic fact that the overwhelming mass of the public were not accustomed to visiting a doctor when they felt well, or were only mildly inconvenienced by a pain or ache. The appeal to the public was not particularly effective because it rested on the assumption that all one has to do is to present the facts and people will draw the expected conclusions, overlooking that human behavior is the result of emotion as well as reason, with the former often more important. The depression and the coming of war also tended to push this topic into the background as other health issues and programs, especially health insurance, became salient. The idea of periodic health examinations lingered on into the thirties and forties, and is still mentioned briefly and condemned with slight praise in the report of President Truman's Commission on the Health Needs of the Nation.[201] But while the periodic health examination did not flourish within the framework of fee-for-service solo practice, it did find a more congenial niche within the environment of prepayment group practice as a preventive service under the concept of comprehensive medical care. With variations, it is an integral part of such plans as Kaiser Permanente, Health Insurance Plan of Greater New York, Group Health Association of Washington, Yale Health Plan and others of the same type serving various populations. The value of such examinations has been the subject of much discussion, but one point is certain; periodic health examinations cannot be performed in any meaningful sense unless there is adequate time for the purpose and the physician has available to him adequate data on the health status of the patient, so that he can arrive at a rational judgment as to any further action on his part, as well as that of the patient. Certainly it is impossible to do so in the situation described by Ward Darley in 1959, when

"patterns of medical care present barriers to the concept of continuing, comprehensive care because of the fragmentation of patient care that has resulted from specialization, practice habits that limit interest to the episodic care of illness, and efficiency measures that limit the amount of time a physician gives to the individual patient."[202]

The negative effect of the structure of medical practice on the provision of preventive services had already been stressed by Wilson G. Smillie over a decade earlier with his comment that "preventive services cannot be effectively incorporated in medical practice unless there is some modification, some change in the present system of payment for medical services in the United States."[203] Thus, about three decades ago, it was clearly recognized that the future of preventive medicine in clinical practice was linked to the organization and financing of health care.

During the thirties, indications began to appear that the established structure of public health was being subjected to critical scrutiny. The issue which evoked this scrutiny was the same problem of medical care. The economic depression, the inception of the New Deal, the final report of the Committee on the Costs of Medical Care, the Social Security Act of 1935—all in one way or another focused attention on the problem of medical care. Within the American Public Health Association this question was being discussed in terms of its relation to public health organization and action.[204] By 1944, the Association had reached a sufficient consensus to adopt an official position set forth in *Medical Care in a National Health Program* which urged that "A national program for medical care should make available to the entire population all essential preventive, diagnostic, and curative services" and "should be adequately and securely financed through social insurance supplemented by general taxation, or by general taxation alone." Four years later a joint statement by the American Public Health Association and the American Hospital Association noted explicitly that "Preventive and curative medicine have reached the stage where they are no longer separable, and it is necessary at the present time to bring them together physically and functionally."[205] Two years later, in 1950, the American Public Health Association adopted a statement of policy on the services and responsibilities of local health departments indicating profound conceptual changes in the nature and scope of public health action:

"As a result of advancing medical knowledge and public health practice, there has been a sharp decrease in morbidity and mortality from infectious diseases, particularly in infancy and childhood and the early years of adult life. Because of the marked changes in the age distribution of the population and in the spectrum of our health problems, the theory and practice of public health has expanded to include not only prevention of the onset of illness, but also prevention of the progress of disease, of associated complications, and of disability and death.

The 'desirable minimum functions' of local health departments—vital statistics, sanitation, communicable disease control, laboratory services, maternal and child health, and health education—have been modified recently to include the control of chronic diseases. Accident prevention, the hygiene of housing, industrial hygiene, school health services, mental health, medical rehabilitation, and hospital and medical care administration are other areas of service and responsibility which have been incorporated into the programs of an increasing number of local health departments."[206]

The full implications of this statement may not have been immediately apparent, but a sense of unease became pervasive in American public health during the fifties and sixties. Symbolic of this situation is the major theme of the annual meeting of the American Public Health Association in 1957, "Is public health in tune with the times?"

In part, this situation was a result of an ambivalent attitude to political action. Departments of public health are creatures of government, and as such the administrators and technical experts who run them are aware of their vulnerability to attack. Furthermore, in reaction to the incompetence fostered by political patronage in official health agencies earlier in the century, American public health developed an "apolitical" stance coupled with an ideology insisting on the elimination of politics from public health work and the elevation of such activities to a professional plane. Public health programs should be judged on the basis of objective, standardized criteria and should not be subjected to arbitrary, individual opinions. Health workers should be recruited and employed on the basis of competence and merit, based on education and training in appropriate schools and apprenticeships, not because of connections or political payoffs. To a very considerable extent these aims have been achieved, but this success has also had unanticipated consequences. As American public health became professionalized, it also tended to become bureaucratic and to insist on strict delimitation of the disciplines involved in it. Furthermore, professionalization tended to turn many public health workers away from public controversy and political battles to what were considered pursuits more appropriate for a professional group, for example, research and demonstration.[207]

To these trends and tendencies must be added a lack of clarity and agreement on objectives, and consequently an absence of realistic and specific programs with which to achieve theoretically desirable goals. This applies specifically to the newer health problems, and the consequent change in the scope and focus of community health activities, which disrupted the previously existing situation and left the diverse groups of health workers without a generally accepted integrated program or a unified institutional structure through which objectives might be realized. The expanding scope of public health brought with it a host of new health workers, thus intensifying the process of specialization which had been going on in organized public health since 1899. In this situation, the centrifugal tendencies inherent in specialization which could be controlled under the earlier arrangements have led to a multiplication of agencies and organizations concerned with health problems. Examples are the separation of mental health activities from public health agencies in numerous instances, the removal of environmental control programs from health departments to other units of government, as well as the ambiguous and not very effective role of public health in dealing with the organization and delivery of personal health services, a major problem of community health.[208]

The same period also saw a massive expansion in medical knowledge derived from research. Immunology, virology, genetics, cytology, biochemistry and molecular biology, all yielded results which could eventually be applied in the prevention of disease. As a result of these developments the conviction has grown that today's health and medical science offered much more than most people got, and that the existing patterns of health service were no longer adequate to deal with current problems.

Certainly there is some justification for this position, as a few examples will illustrate. An entirely new way of thinking about non-hereditary anomalies was opened up by N.McA. Gregg's study of an outbreak of congenital cataract among Australian newborns during 1940-41, most of whom also had cardiac, auditory, dental and other defects. Gregg advanced the hypothesis, since amply confirmed, that maternal infection with rubella accounted for the increased prevalence of congenital defects among these infants. The seriousness of this problem is revealed by the fact that the peak of the last epidemic cycle of rubella caused severe birth defects among more than 20,000 American children. Today, rubella vaccine, available since 1969, can be used to immunize children aged one to nine, as well as susceptible women of childbearing age. As a result, the number of reported cases of rubella has been greatly reduced and there is less chance for pregnant women to be exposed. Also abortion is more easily available to women who have been exposed.[209]

Similarly, knowledge and techniques are presently available to prevent hemolytic disease of the newborn as well as to reduce greatly the incidence of mental retardation. With respect to the former, studies of feedback mechanisms governing antibody synthesis led eventually to a method for prevention of Rh immunization by giving small doses of anti-Rh to Rh negative women. Widespread use of this method would probably eradicate this disease and eliminate about 7,500 cases annually in the United States.[210]

Mental retardation or deficiency is the result of several different causes. Some such as Down's syndrome are inherited, others are congenital and are due to infections, such as rubella, or other noxious agents. At present, a number of possibilities exist for prevention. As Zena Stein points out these include "the discovery of parents who are carriers of recessive genes, birth control, amniocentesis and induced abortion, screening at birth and treatment, and intensive enrichment programs in early childhood."[211] Application of currently available knowledge would eliminate about 30 percent of severe retardation and a larger proportion of milder forms.

Prophylaxis is now possible for the 20,000 Americans who are afflicted with hemophilia. The isolation of an antihemophiliac factor which can be administered two or three times weekly to those afflicted with this condition has made it possible for such persons to carry on most ordinary activities including sports.[212]

The introduction and use of various drugs has made it possible to control diseases which previously severely incapacitated and soon killed their victims. One example is hypertensive heart disease. Beginning around 1940, the mortality rates for hypertensive heart disease declined with a steeper rate of decline developing early in the 1950s. The decline has been greater for whites than for non-whites. Why a decline occurred from 1940 to 1950 is not known. Whether this development was the result of biological or social processes operating alone or in combination remains a problem for investigation. However, the steeper downward trend that appeared in the 1950s and continued thereafter was due in large part to the introduction of drugs which effectively lowered blood pressure (hexamethonium, hydralazine, rauwolfia and methyldopa). The varying experience of whites and non-whites may be due in some measure to biological factors, but the role of socio-economic factors, including inadequate medical care, is much more important for control.[213]

An earlier instance of this kind is the introduction of insulin in 1922 and later that of tolbutamide. Although there has been no dramatic change in the death rate from diabetes, these drugs have made it increasingly possible for diabetics to live longer, as well as to be productive and comfortable. Records at the Joslin Clinic reveal that patients who were first examined and treated within one year after the onset of illness had a more favorable survivorship experience than those whose disease was diagnosed and treated later. Other data indicate that the average duration of life after the onset of diabetes has increased greatly particularly for diabetics under twenty.[214] What this indicates is the necessity for early diagnosis and treatment.

There are, of course, other new drugs which are being used to control epilepsy, parkinsonism, asthma, and mental and emotional conditions. The use of such pharmacologic agents and their consequences cannot be discussed here, but the tendency for such intervention to increase must be kept in mind as an aspect of current and future disease prevention and control. In practically all diseases of this kind, knowledge of the precise factors that lead to the onset of disease are inadequate, even though epidemiological, clinical and other studies may have elucidated some factors that are involved. For example, it is known that there is a genetic element in the occurrence of diabetes, but whether or not a given individual will develop diabetes cannot be predicted with certainty. Nevertheless, such knowledge can raise the physician's level of suspicion and alert him to the possible existence of disease in persons with an appropriate family history. In short, in the absence of knowledge on which primary prevention might be based, one must have recourse to detection of possible candidates for diagnosis and treatment. The achievement of this aim presupposes some mechanism by which such persons could be brought to the attention of health personnel. A number of such structures are already in existence, for example, neighborhood health centers, group practice units, hospital centers, health department clinics, industrial health facilities, health plans in educational institutions, and the like. At present these are more or less isolated entities. A future aim with respect to disease prevention and control is to see how they might be linked in a national network, perhaps as part of a national health insurance plan.

On the other hand, in some non-communicable diseases, the etiology and the pathogenetic process have been largely elucidated, and yet for social and economic reasons relatively little has been done to prevent or to control the problem. Two examples are dental caries and lung cancer.

Based on the work of McKay, Dean, Cox and others, there is now enough evidence to show unequivocally that ingestion of water-borne fluoride can reduce dental caries by as much as 60 percent. Moreover, controlled water fluoridation has been shown to be safe. Nevertheless, this practice has not been accepted by a considerable number of local communities and in some has been accepted only after bitter conflicts. Fluoridation began about 1950 and by 1964 more than 2,600 communities with about 47 million people had fluoridated water supplies. Of the 50 largest cities in the United States, in 1960, 21 were using controlled fluoridated water and two had naturally fluoridated water. By 1967, over 3000 communities with a total population of 60 million people had adopted fluoridation. Since then there has been some improvement in the situation, but the controversy over water fluoridation has not completely abated. A great deal of effort still has to be exerted to provide optimally fluoridated drinking water to all populations with piped water systems.

By 1964, a causal relationship between smoking, particularly cigarette smoking and the occurrence of lung cancer had been sufficiently well established for the U.S. Public Health Service to issue its first report on *Smoking and Health*, warning of the hazards associated with this practice. Nevertheless, despite repeated efforts to have people stop smoking, whether by persuasion, scare tactics, or other means, no large measure of success has been attained. There are probably just as many smokers, if not more, today as there were in 1964. Reasons for this failure are evident; they are social, economic and psychological. Many young people begin to smoke because this behavior symbolizes adulthood, and are confirmed in its appropriateness by peer group approval. The tobacco industry panders to the market available among young people by associating the pleasures of smoking with nature, romance, glamour, adventure and other presumably attractive and gratifying aspects of early adulthood. Moreover, the resources of this industry far outweigh those available to the opponents of smoking, chiefly voluntary and professional agencies, as well as official health agencies to a lesser extent. Political and economic constraints have so far hindered any serious legislative action at the federal level. As a result, in this situation, where primary prevention by cessation or avoidance of smoking would seem to be the method of choice, it has been necessary to accept the unpalatable fact that this aim cannot be achieved by a frontal attack. The methods employed at present comprise public education on a limited scale, informing smokers of the tar and nicotine content of cigarettes by placing this information on the package, endeavoring to restrict smoking in public places, and providing clinics for those who find it difficult to give up smoking. These measures plus increased taxation on tobacco products, particularly cigarettes were proposed in 1962 by the Royal College of Physicians of London, but so far do not seem to have been effectual.[215]

Whether such measures will be any more effective in the future is doubtful, as long as no account is taken of the relation of smoking to culturally conditioned patterns of behavior of which it is a part. The role of cultural conditioning in the formation of food habits has been recognized for some time, and has led to an awareness that any endeavor to change eating patterns must take this basic fact into account. Furthermore, people will change their food habits when such a change seems relevant to their concerns. For example, a growing interest in so-called natural foods, as well as health concerns of persons over 40, seem to have contributed to a decline in coffee drinking and an increase in the consumption of decaffeinated coffee.[216] Perhaps the production of an acceptable denicotinized cigarette will help solve the problem of lung cancer due to smoking.

Deaths and injuries due to accidents can also be reduced, though here too there are economic and institutional barriers. That prevention can be practiced is evident from the experience with occupational accidents over the past 50 years. Despite a greatly expanded labor force, deaths of workers on the job were reduced from 19,000 in 1928 to 13,800 in 1960. The work accident rate in 1960, 22 deaths per 100,000 workers, was just half of the rate in 1937, 43 per 100,000. Much of this decline is the result of improvements in working conditions, the installation of proper safety devices for automatic machinery, the use of protective devices by workers, better medical care for workers, safety legislation, and a variety of safety campaigns. The role of workmen's compensation and the enlightened self-interest of employers in certain industries has also been significant. Some industries such as mining continue to be extremely hazardous, but here too the application of available knowledge and techniques can effectively reduce the toll of dead and injured workers.[217]

Since the beginning of the century mortality from all accidents has declined when measured against the growth of population. Nevertheless, accidents continue to rank high among the leading causes of death in the United States. In 1960 and more recently, accidents have been exceeded only by heart disease, cancer and cerebrovascular lesions. This situation has resulted from the declines in the mortality of the major communicable diseases combined with a rise in deaths due to motor vehicle accidents. That the latter can also be prevented is indicated by experience since the need to conserve energy resources led to a reduced speed limit of 50 miles per hour, and the rise in the price of gasoline tended to diminish the volume of traffic somewhat. Since then there has been a noticeable decline in the number of accidents, deaths and injuries. Furthermore, even if accidents are not avoided, it is still possible to prevent injury or death by altering the environment. Roadside guardrails, for example, can be quite effective in this respect. Prevention does not necessarily require a complete understanding of all the factors involved in the causation of disease or injury. All that is necessary is that the effectiveness of the preventive measure match the objective to be achieved.[218]

This applies particularly to a disease such as cancer. Primary prevention can be practiced where workers in certain industries are exposed to carcinogenic substances, for example radioactive ores, chromates, asbestos, or aniline dyes. But such exposures represent only a relatively minor element in the etiology of most cancers. The fact of the matter is that available knowledge on which to base primary prevention is very limited. For this reason the only available option is to practice secondary prevention, that is, detection of the disease at an early stage so as to prevent progression and increase length of life. At present, for example, there is no explanation for the continued declining trend in the incidence as well as the mortality of stomach cancer.[219] Or why the incidence and mortality of cancer of the pancreas have been increasing.

On the other hand, there is evidence that the morbidity and mortality of cervical cancer have been declining over the past two decades, and that this trend may be due to the use of cytologic screening. Within several years after the announcement by George Papanicolaou in 1941 of the diagnostic value of vaginal smears in the detection of uterine cancer, this technique began to be applied for screening.[220] Recently, Daniel Cramer has pointed to a positive correlation between the rate of cytologic screening and the decrease in the morbidity and mortality of cervical cancer, indicating the possibility of a causal role for the screening technique.[221] Though this conclusion may be disputed, a recent report on the subject agreed that "cytologic screening is an important tool in the prevention and control of cancer of the uterine cervix."[222] Similarly, the use of screening techniques for breast cancer, particularly self-examination and mammography, have been found useful. There are problems connected with most screening methods, but there is little doubt that secondary prevention through detection, diagnosis and therapy are at present the best available means for cancer control.[223]

A recent study by the National Center for Health Statistics revealed that over the twenty years from 1950 to 1969, the age adjusted death rates for heart disease dropped by 15 percent. Why this occurred is an unanswered question. Nevertheless, one may note that hypertensive disease is a major factor increasing the risk of coronary heart disease, and since the mortality trend among whites has declined, it may have had an effect on heart disease mortality. Another factor may be the decreasing incidence of rheumatic fever in children and consequently of chronic rheumatic heart disease. Still these are only hypotheses. With respect to coronary heart disease, J.N. Morris asserts

> "there is no proof in the conventional sense that by altering behavior in accord with the results of observational studies which have been carried out—controlling weight, abandoning cigarettes, taking adequate exercise, or lowering blood pressure and lipid values in middle age—individual risk and population incidence will be lowered."[224]

In the face of this conclusion, Morris falls back on a counsel which derives from antiquity and which was already traditional when it was incorporated in the medieval Regimen of Health of Salerno, that is, to maintain health by living moderately, by regulating diet, exercise, emotional stress and other aspects of life. If this is not a counsel of despair, it is at least a recognition that an adequate basis for prevention of coronary heart disease is not presently available.

Obviously, the situation with respect to many of the important current health problems—the non-communicable chronic diseases—is analogous to the state of affairs around 1870 in terms of understanding and preventing the communicable diseases. What then is to be done? Whither preventive medicine?

Whither Preventive Medicine?

Obviously it is not possible to give a detailed blueprint of things to come. There are, however, several points to be considered in terms of trends, and we may do so by using a statement prepared in 1951 by an international group of experts under the sponsorship of the World Health Organization. "Modern public health," they said,

> "has been developed during the last hundred years from primarily a legislative and police function to an applied science, which constitutes an important and integral part of social and economic evolution. The techniques used in health administration have consequently been changed to emphasize positive measures in planning and organizing the modern health services on a community basis, in order to create a healthy environment for the people, and in educating the public for active participation in health work."[225] .

In the United States, the situation which existed throughout the first half of the century has disintegrated during the past 25 years. The relatively simple division between prevention and cure in terms of official and voluntary health agencies on the one hand, clinical practitioners on the other, has vanished. Today this situation has dissolved into a multiplicity of organizations all involved in some way with disease prevention and control. Clearly this is a transition period, in which new arrangements for community health services are being developed. In this situation the need for policy guidelines to achieve coordination among agencies is essential. Efforts have been made to develop such a policy through the creation of a National Commission on Community Health Services in 1962 sponsored by the American Public Health Association and the National Health Council. From the final report of the Commission, *Health is a Community Affair* (1966), it is clear that the sharp lines of responsibility that once characterized the activities of official health agencies have been broken down, specifically with respect to the distinction between prevention and cure, and that there is a clear need for a single system of care for the provision of personal health services. Vaious steps taken on a national level during the last decade may also be seen as tentative and hesitant moves toward a national health policy and the creation of a unified system to provide health care for all. Medicare, Medicaid, neighborhood health centers, community mental health centers—all represent some effort in this direction, no matter now limited, as do the two federally sponsored efforts at reorganizing and rationalizing the health care delivery system, that is, comprehensive health planning and regional medical programs. But to paraphrase and amend Galileo, though it does move, there is still a long way to go. Comprehensive health planning and regional medical programs can only be described as embryonic, and all the other programs had their troubles.

These programs were replaced in 1974 by the National Health Policy, Planning and Resources Development Act. The passage of this legislation is the most recent stage in a process which began over 40 years ago, and which has been moving the United States toward a national system of interrelated local, state and Federal health planning. In all likelihood, the 1974 Act will have an important impact on future activities and programs for health maintenance and disease prevention.

The origins of this evolution are to be found in the period of the thirties when few hospitals were built due to the financial difficulties of the depression. Because of the same situation, existing facilities tended to deteriorate and become obsolete so that by the end of the Second World War there was a marked shortage of hospital beds. This problem was further aggravated by maldistribution of facilities and beds among the states and between urban and rural areas. To identify precisely and to deal with the deficiencies, Senators Hill and Burton introduced the Hospital Survey and Construction Act, which was enacted into law in 1946 and provided the basis for the Hill-Burton program. This was the first step toward effective health planning and resources development on a national basis.

Initially, each state received a grant to survey its needs for hospitals and other health care facilities, and to prepare a plan to meet them. Following federal approval of the plan, funds were allotted to carry out a construction program. Although the original program was subsequently extended and slightly expanded, it experienced little change until 1964 when the Hill-Burton Act was modified by the addition of legislative authority for funding area-wide planning councils for health facilities. These councils were generally made up of community leaders and providers of health care, and were intended to plan the development of needed hospitals and other health facilities for their area or region on a continuing basis. This program was soon criticized, however, on the ground that it had a built-in bias toward expensive health facilities, and that what was needed was a more comprehensive approach which would consider in the planning process not only physical facilities but also health personnel, services and other programs and activities with an influence on the people's health. To deal with these shortcomings, the Comprehensive Health Planning and Public Health Services Amendments were enacted in 1966, and modified the following year by the Partnership for Health Amendments. Additional changes were made in 1970. The agencies authorized by this legislation were given a broad mandate to plan for all aspects of the health system in the area which they covered. Eventually the make-up of the governing councils of the agencies was spelled out to include governmental, institutional, professional and community representation. In addition, a National Advisory Council on Comprehensive Health Planning Programs was established to advise on policy matters relating to health planning. Then, in 1972, the concept that health planning and health financing should be closely related was embodied in section 1122 of the Social Security Act.

Paralleling this development since 1965 and eventually converging with it has been the evolution of the Regional Medical Programs, which grew out of the Report of the President's Commission on Heart Disease, Cancer and Stroke, published in December, 1964. The Report proposed "the establishment of a national network of Regional Heart Disease, Cancer and Stroke Centers for clinical investigation, teaching and patient care, in universities, hospitals and research institutes and other institutions across the country."[226] However, in response to objections from medical practitioners who were concerned that the regional medical centers would be dominated by academic medicine, the legislation enacted in 1965 authorized regional cooperative arrangements among health care institutions, medical schools and research establishments as the means for making available to patients suffering from heart disease, cancer or stroke the best diagnostic and therapeutic care. In 1970, the categorical disease focus was slightly expanded by the inclusion of kidney diseases. In addition, the regional programs were linked to comprehensive health planning agencies in that the latter could review and comment on grant proposals affecting their planning areas. There was also an emphasis on primary care linking it to secondary and tertiary care. In 1973, the regional program would have been allowed to lapse, had not the Congress extended it to 1974.

The Act of 1974 fused the three earlier programs (Hill-Burton, Comprehensive Health Planning, and Regional Medical Programs) into a unitary system for national health planning and development with guidelines and priorities. In the formulation of health goals, "the promotion of activities for the prevention of disease, including studies of nutritional and environmental factors affecting health and the provision of preventive health care services." Another priority is "the development of effective methods of educating the general public concerning proper personal (including preventive) health care and methods for effective use of available health services."

This is clearly a mandate for a preventive program to include health maintenance, disease prevention, and health education. Existing programs and activities must be concentrated in these areas, while at the same time new knowledge must be developed and evaluated so that it can be applied for the benefit of the American people. Specific proposals to develop and to implement these general objectives have been set forth in the *Forward Plan for 1976-1980*. Through such activities as well as through intensive educational work among medical and other health personnel, prevention can be given the place in the health arena which its importance deserves. In this respect the *Forward Plan* requires careful study.

The current pattern of education for public health workers was initiated when the School of Hygiene and Public Health at Johns Hopkins was opened on October 1, 1918, and set a pattern for others to follow. As of December, 1974, there were 19 schools of public health accredited by the Council on Education for Public Health, including one in Canada. Historically their emergence can be classified in three phases: the period up to the First World War, the period between the two world wars, and the period after the Second World War. The first schools of public health appeared, as we have seen, in response to the movement for the professionalization of public health work, chiefly in official health agencies. This trend was furthered from two directions. The movement to establish local health units had been developing for almost a decade before the first school was created at Johns Hopkins. Under the stimulation and guidance, and with the assistance of a number of organizations, county health work developed and expanded between 1910 and 1940. Among the organizations which took an early and prominent part were the U.S. Public Health Service and the Rockefeller Foundation. The Milbank Fund and the Commonwealth Fund contributed a further impetus through their demonstrations.[227] These and other health organizations worked with state health departments to induce county authorities to organize, finance and administer local health service. The depression years undoubtedly retarded this development, and budgets for organized county health units remained low. As a result, physicians were not attracted because of inadequate renumeration, and equally important because of insufficient opportunity for professional growth.

This tendency was in part overcome by another factor. The role of government in relation to health had been increasing during the first three decades of the century. However, with the enactment of the Social Security Act of 1935 the role of the federal government entered upon a new stage of development which was to have important consequences for public health and preventive medicine. For example, the Act carried the Maternity and Infancy Act further by authorizing grants to be made each year to the various states through the Children's Bureau to help them extend and improve their maternal and child health services, as well as those for handicapped children. Steps were also taken within this context to advance nutrition services. Industrial hygiene was another health area stimulated by the Social Security Act, and additional efforts were undertaken to provide more local health units. The creation of programs and agencies increased the need for personnel, so that funds made available through grants-in-aid greatly stimulated the education and training of public health workers. As a result, during the period from 1920 to 1950, the students who attended the schools of public health had some connection with official health agencies. The majority of the students were persons already holding positions in health departments who needed academic instruction and perhaps supervised field training to improve and broaden their professional competence. A smaller group were newcomers,

72

but most of them would also join official health agencies. Furthermore, a very large proportion of the students were physicians. Thus, by the 1940s, there existed a group of physicians specially trained in public health and preventive medicine, but whose professional status was low in comparison with that of private clinical practitioners. This state of affairs became particularly galling during the Second World War when physicians trained in preventive medicine were not identified and treated as specialists.

The first step toward improving this situation was taken in 1948-49 with the establishment of the American Board of Preventive Medicine and Public Health. At the beginning the Board dealt with the certification of specialists in public health. In 1952, however, the term "Public Health" was dropped from the Board's title and over the next eight years three more specialty groups were added—aviation medicine, 1953, occupational medicine, 1955, and general preventive medicine, 1960. These events were followed by the development of residency programs on the pattern of the hospital-based specialties, though the residencies were in health agencies for the most part.[228] The establishment of the Board was also followed in 1954 by the creation of the American College of Preventive Medicine as an organizational center for the new specialty, to represent its interests and to foster its development.

The establishment of the American Board of Preventive Medicine and of the American College of Preventive Medicine was intended to deal with the problem by raising the prestige of this group of physicians and thereby attract new recruits to the field. Although this situation has improved somewhat in the past two decades, the problems still exist, and in some respect have become intensified. During this period, preventive medicine has been undergoing a transition comparable to that being experienced by public health, and in both cases for the same reasons, basically the altered character and locale of the prevalent health problems in the United States, as well as the changed social factors to which they are related.

The 1950s and 1960s brought sharp changes to the health scene with an increased emphasis, as described above, on the chronic diseases with their more complex and in varying degrees unknown etiologies, their lengthy period of development, and the major involvement of middle-aged and older adults. For the schools of public health this has led to changes in their curricula and in the composition of the faculties and the student bodies. Emphasis has been placed on epidemiology, including its methodology; biostatistics; health organization and administration, including medical care; environmental health in its recent aspects, thus incorporating occupational health, health education and behavioral science; as well as various aspects of international health among them demography and population problems. This process of reorientation, which is by no means ended, occurred during a period of expansion. Between 1950 and 1970, the number of schools of public health in the United States doubled. Faculties were enlarged and diversified. National legislation authorizing federal funding for both training and research (Hill-Rhodes, general and special purpose traineeships, *et alia*) provided financial support through the Department of Health, Education and Welfare, and more particularly through the National Institutes of Health, and the schools of public health secured the necessary funding for the instruction of students, as well as for research and community demonstration projects. The legislation of 1965-66, including Medicare, Medicaid, Comprehensive Health Planning and Regional Medical Programs added a further thrust to the explosive expansion of this period.

One major aspect of the change effected by these developments is the changed character of the students and their professional goals. As a consequence of traineeship support many students without prior public health experience entered the schools. A large number of these students did not look toward future employment only in official or voluntary health agencies, but wished to embark on careers in administration, service and research in medical care, health insurance, environmental problems and other areas that were being defined. The impact of federal support for training is most evident in the output of graduates who can work in fields of high sociomedical saliency, and provides a most emphatic argument for the future continuation of such support.

The situation in medical schools with respect to departments of preventive medicine is not identical but analogous (the term "preventive medicine" as employed in this connection stands also for various other designations such as "community medicine"). The curriculum content of these units as it existed before the Second World War has changed because of the medical and social problems requiring preventive action. Furthermore, the health field like other aspects of our society is governed in many ways by a market structure and mentality. If the incentives toward preventive medicine were to outweigh whatever presumed disadvantages exist, more physicians would undoubtedly be interested. As long as private clinical practice is considered more rewarding financially and in terms of professional status, preventive medicine will be at the end of the procession. Federal training support can be important in providing incentives as it has done in schools of public health. At the same time, it is also important to show medical students that preventive medicine has a scientific basis in such disciplines as epidemiology, pathology, biostatistics, demography and biochemistry. Yet as Michael M. Davis observed, "There is no public health, only individual health." In this sense, the department of preventive medicine can bridge the gap between the health problems of individuals and the health concerns of the larger group. This can perhaps be accomplished by linking the teaching of preventive medicine to selected clinical .fields, e.g. internal medicine, pediatrics, and obstetrics-gynecology. In working out such patterns the American College of Preventive

Medicine should play a central role. But these are questions that can only be raised here, not solved.

Nevertheless, some benchmarks have been established, a beginning has been made, and there are indications for possible future evolution. As such institutional forms are developed they will provide the context for the practice of preventive medicine. However, their creation and organization will require planning, which in turn requires health intelligence. According to Karl Evang, what is needed is

"careful, long-term planning based upon epidemiological research instead of swiftly improvised solutions, minute weighing of priorities in relation to available resources, coordination to avoid overlapping and duplication of effort, and analysis of methods and assessments of results."[229]

Health intelligence is meaningful, however, only if it is applied, and this can be done most fruitfully and effectively within a community setting. Leadership and organization in the promotion of health, in preventive medicine, in calling attention to health problems have all been functions of public health in the past and can be in the future. This does not mean, however, that all personal health services have to be provided by official health agencies. This has not been the case in the past, nor can it be in the future. The future of public health is in the development of a community health service in which its major functions should be collection and analysis of demographic data, surveillance of disease and epidemiological investigations, standard setting, regulation and inspection, and provision of services where these are required but do not exist.

In the last analysis, the functions of official health agencies depend on the scope permitted them by the legislative bodies from whom they derive their powers and funds. For this reason a large measure of the preventive service will probably be provided by other organizations and groups, among them group practices, health maintenance organizations, neighborhood health centers, industrial clinics, screening centers and detection clinics associated with hospitals. However, these entities should be elements within a larger health care delivery system for which experience gained so far in comprehensive health planning and regional medical programs can be useful. Emphasis must be placed on coordination of services, since detection of noncommunicable diseases is meaningless unless there is follow-up for diagnosis and treatment, as well as follow-up thereafter as required. This aspect must be seen in the light of the fact that a very large part of our population, perhaps 20 percent or more, receives its ambulatory medical care through emergency rooms or hospital based outpatient clinics, and this care tends to be episodic and not infrequently symptomatic.[230] Finally, the context in which these services will be provided and their financing are probably going to be determined by the kind of health insurance system the United

States will have in the immediate future, perhaps through the next decade. If it will follow the current arrangements of voluntary health insurance, Medicare and Medicaid, the outlook for preventive services may be dim. On the other hand, if the emphasis will be on comprehensive service in a coordinated system such as group practice, the outlook will be more promising. In any event, if past experience is any guide, the outcome is likely to be a compromise, but those interested in the provision of preventive services should work for a coordinated system rather than a fragmented one such as we have at present. Moreover, a coordinated system would be able to make better use of paramedical personnel who are very likely going to loom larger in the medical practice of the future.

From the description provided above, it should be clear that the new preventive medicine which begain to emerge only about 25 years ago is still only in its beginnings. For the most part it is based on epidemiological studies combined with laboratory and clinical investigations. In the future, knowledge for prevention will continue to be derived from epidemiology, but one must note that such studies have limitations. In numerous instances, they are based on statistical analyses, and can report only on correlations that point to possible etiological factors, but cannot provide a basis for action. For this reason, close cooperation with clinical investigators and greater emphasis on clinical epidemiology as advocated by John R. Paul is in order for future research in preventive medicine. A model of how clinical data, social epidemiology and laboratory investigation can be combined is available in the classic work of Goldberger on pellagra. This is the type of research which can be carried on by departments of preventive medicine in medical schools and by schools of public health. Moreover, the use of such studies in teaching and possibly the involvement of students in research projects may make preventive medicine more acceptable in the medical school environment.

The continuing need for various forms of prevention developed in the earlier history of preventive medicine cannot seriously be questioned. Maternal and child health must continue to receive attention though the areas of concern have changed greatly since the beginning of the century. Child development in its various aspects is the major focus of preventive interest for the future. As long as communicable diseases are controlled because the population at risk is immunized, then specific primary prevention of this type must be continued at a level appropriate to the particular disease. Failure to immunize infants and children against diphtheria, poliomyelitis or any of the other communicable diseases for which specific protection is available, simply means that outbreaks can be expected as soon as the necessary conditions are present. Moreover, immunization against rubella is also a way of preventing congenital defects in the infants of mothers exposed to the disease. The same may be said of pasteurization, sanitation of water and food, the control of air pollution and in general various aspects of the environment which may have a deleterious influence on health. This is particularly relevant as new products and processes become a part of the environment of the producer and the consumer. The occupational environment should be a subject of major interest for preventive medicine. This should also be the case with mental and emotional health, an area in which there is very little solid knowledge on which to base preventive action.

As long as means of primary prevention do not exist, and until greater clarity and more knowledge are available for various chronic diseases, secondary prevention through detection, diagnosis and treatment should be pursued by such means as are feasible and effective, for example, cytologic screening, glaucoma detection, mammography and others. For such an approach to be effective it will have to be used with more precise knowledge of groups at risk and evaluation of findings. This also requires as far as possible the establishment of the natural history of the particular disease. All these aspects are obviously subjects for research.

Finally, attention must be called again to the socio-economic environment and its relation to disease prevention and control. Although proper living and working conditions will not necessarily prevent all disease, there is no doubt that good housing, proper nutrition, absence of undue emotional stress, suitable working conditions, provision of mental stimulation and physical recreation are more likely to produce a healthy people, than poverty, malnutrition, ignorance, decrepit housing and the other social evils that are associated with ill health. We have seen how a disease such as tuberculosis has evolved as a result of a biosocial process extending over a number of years. Quite possibly similar developments are occurring with respect to heart disease and gastric cancer. In any event, the future of preventive medicine is bright if one can envisage it as in the early stages of a period which only began about 25 or 30 years ago and is likely to continue along the lines indicated well into the twenty-first century. A hundred years ago the pioneers of preventive medicine who began to control communicable diseases could not foresee what the outcome of their efforts would be, nor can we do so with respect to today's problems. Yet this should not stop us from continuing the odyssey of preventive medicine, for its interest and fascination spring from the unknown that awaits us.

References

[1] Albert J. Mayer, "Life Expectancy in the City of Chicago 1880–1950," *Human Biology* 27:202–210 (1955).

[2] U.S. Department of Health, Education and Welfare, *Toward A Social Report*, with an introductory commentary by Wilbur J. Cohen (Ann Arbor, University of Michigan Press, 1970), pp. 1–2.

[3] George M. Kober, *Report of the Committee on Social Betterment*, (Washington, D.C., President's Homes Commission, 1908), pp. 59–60; Monroe Lerner and Odin W. Anderson, *Health Progress in the United States 1900–1960* (Chicago, Ill., University of Chicago Press, 1963), pp. 14–16; Carl C. Dauer, Robert F. Korns and Leonard M. Schuman, *Infectious Diseases* (Cambridge, Mass., Harvard University Press, 1968), p. 1.

[4] Edgar Sydenstricker, "The Vitality of the American People," in *Recent Social Trends in the United States. Report of the President's Research Committee on Social Trends* (New York, McGraw-Hill, 1933), p. 630.

[5] Grover F. Powers, "Developments in Pediatrics in the Past Quarter Century," *Yale J. Biol. & Med.* 12:1–22 (1939) (see p. 9).

[6] *Ibid.*, p. 8; Borden S. Veeder, *Preventive Pediatrics* (New York, D. Appleton & Co., 1926), p. 147.

[7] William Osler, *Principles and Practice of Medicine*, 4th edition (Edinburgh and London, Young J. Pentland, 1901), p. 434; also see St. Engel and Grete Katzenstein, "Versuch einer Morbiditätsstatistik der Rachitis," *Archiv für Kinderheilkunde* 70:198–212 (1922); Franz Wiltschke, "Ergebnisse einer Rachitisuntersuchung in Graz," *Archiv für Kinderheilkunde* 74:241–255 (1924).

[8] E.V. McCollum, "Nutrition as a Factor in Physical Development," *Annals of the American Academy of Political and Social Science* 98:34–43 (1921).

[9] National Health Insurance. Medical Research Committee. *A Study of Social and Economic Factors in The Causation of Rickets* by Margaret Ferguson, with *an Introductory Historical Survey*, by Leonard Findlay (London, H.M.S.O., 1918), p. 97; George Newman, *An Outline of the Practice of Preventive Medicine. A Memorandum addressed to the Minister of Health* (London, H.M.S.O., 1919), pp. 79–80.

[10] Elmer Verner McCollum, *From Kansas Farm Boy to Scientist* (Lawrence, University of Kansas Press, 1964), pp. 165–171; Edward Mellanby, *Experimental Rickets* (Medical Research Council) (London, H.M.S.O., 1921).

[11] Robert Hunter, *Poverty* (New York, Macmillan, 1904), p. 216.

[12] John Spargo, *The Bitter Cry of the Children* (New York, 1906), pp. 1–124.

[13] J.A. Saltzman, *Principles and Practice of Public Health Dentistry* (Boston, Stratford Co., 1937), p. 65.

[14] R.C. Chapin, *The Standard of Living Among Workingmen's Families in New York City* (New York, Russell Sage Foundation, 1909), p. 190.

[15] *Report of the Health Insurance Commission of the State of Illinois, May, 1919* (Springfield, Ill., Illinois State Journal Co., 1919), p. 17.

[16] J.M. Slemons, "Progress in Obstetrics: 1890-1940," *Amer. J. Surg.*, n.s., 51:83–84 (1941).

[17]R.W. Bruère, "A Plan for the Reduction of Infant Mortality," *Bull. Am. Acad. Med.* 11:261 (1910).

[18]Michael M. Davis, *Immigrant Health and the Community* (New York, Harper & Bros., 1921), p. 196; John A. Ferrell, "The Trend of Preventive Medicine in the United States," *J.A.M.A.* 81:1063–1069 (1923) (see p. 22).

[19]Anna E. Rude, "The Midwife Problem in the United States," *J.A.M.A.* 81:987–992 (1923).

[20]J.H. Larson, "A Maternity and Infant Welfare Program for the United States," *Amer. J. Pub. Health* 8:483–484 (1918).

[21]Dorothy E. Bradbury, *Four Decades of Action for Children. A Short History of the Children's Bureau* (Children's Bureau Publication No. 358) (Washington, D.C., Govt. Printing Office, 1956), p. 7.

[22]S.J. Baker, "The Reduction of Infant Mortality in New York City," *Amer. J. Dis. Child.* 5:151, 158–159 (1913).

[23]For a detailed account of the beginnings of occupational health in the United States and their relation to developments in Europe and Great Britain see George Rosen: *A History of Public Health* (New York, M.D. Publications, 1958), pp. 419–439.

[24]Alice Hamilton, *Exploring the Dangerous Trades* (Boston, Little, Brown and Co., 1943), p. 128.

[25]Henry W. Farnam, "Introductory Address," *First National Conference on Industrial Diseases, Chicago, June 10, 1910* (American Association for Labor Legislation, Publication No. 10) (New York, American Association for Labor Legislation, 1910), pp. 5–6. The Association had been founded in 1906 and existed until 1942. Farnam was professor of economics at Yale University from 1880 to 1918, and a founder of the Association as well as its president during its first four years. He had a major interest in social legislation, and his last work, published posthumously, was *Chapters in the History of Social Legislation in the United States to 1860* (Washington, D.C., Carnegie Institution, 1938).

[26]Rosen, *op. cit.*, p. 428.

[27]W.C. Garrison, *Health Conditions of the Pottery Industry. The Eight Hour Movement. Wages and Production in the Glass Industry. 1905* (Monograph on Economic Subjects. From the Twenty-Eighth Annual Report of the Bureau of Statistics of New Jersey), n.d. (1905?), pp. 107–127.

[28]J.W. Schereschewsky *The Health of Garment Workers* (Public Health Bulletin No. 71. Studies in Vocational Diseases) (Washington, G.P.O., 1915), pp. 13–103.

[29]George M. Kober, *Industrial and Personal Hygiene. A Report of the Committee on Social Betterment* (Washington, President's Homes Commission, 1908). J.H. Lloyd in 1902 had written on "The Diseases of Occupation" for the system *Twentieth Century Practice of Medicine*, but it was not as comprehensive as Kober's book. For Kober see George Rosen, "From Frontier Surgeon to Industrial Hygienist: The Strange Career of George M. Kober," *Amer. J. Publ. Health* 65:638–643 (1975).

[30]Evidence of this trend may be seen in the growing volume of publications, reports, books, articles in periodicals, pamphlets and the like, that appeared during the period 1910–1925. The following publications are only a small sample: New York State Department of Labor Industrial Board, *Rules relating to the Removal of Dust, Gases*

and *Fumes*, Bulletin No. 12 (New York City, 1915); R.J. Sewall, "Caisson-Disease on the Cuyuna Iron Range," *Journal-Lancet* (Minn.) (May 15, 1915), pp. 3–26; "Spray-process hazards," *The Travelers Standard* 5:187–192 (1917); Gordon L. Berry, *Eye Hazards in Industrial Occupations. A Report of Typical Cases and Conditions, with Recommendations for Safe Practice*, (New York, National Committee for the Prevention of Blindness, 1917); David Van Schaack, *Accident Prevention in Textile Plants*, An Address given at Boston, Mass., February 14, 1918, during the Seventh Annual Conference of Lockwood, Greene & Co., (n.p., n.d.); "Proposed Employment of Women during the War in the Industries of Niagara Falls, N.Y.," *Monthly Labor Review* (January, 1919), pp. 231–245; *Hours of Work as Related to Output and Health of Workers. Silk Manufacturing Research Report* No. 16 (National Industrial Conference Board, March 1919); Agnes de Lima, *Night-Working Mothers in Textile Mills. Passaic, New Jersey* (National Consumer's League); Consumers League of New Jersey, December, 1920; *Health Facts in Support of the Five-Day Week for Painters. Report prepared by the Workers' Health Bureau, including an analysis by Dr. Emery R. Hayhurst. . . of the medical records of 267 New York painters examined in the Journeymen Painters and Allied Crafts Health Department*, issued by New York District Council No. 9, Brotherhood of Painters, Decorators and Paperhangers of America (New York, Workers' Health Bureau, 1923); C.-E.A. Winslow, "Industrial Tuberculosis," *Bulletin New York Tuberculosis Association* 6:1, 5–7 (1925); Louis I. Harris, "Tuberculosis and Industry," *ibid.* 6:7–9 (1925); Arthur L. Murray, *Lead Poisoning in the Mining of Lead in Utah* (Technical Paper 389, Bureau of Mines) (Washington, G.P.O., 1926); Rollo H. Britten and L.R. Thompson, *A Health Study of Ten Thousand Male Industrial Workers* (Public Health Bulletin No. 162) (Washington, D.C., G.P.O., 1926).

[31] George M. Kober, *Industrial and Personal Hygiene. A Report of the Committee on Social Betterment* (Washington, D.C., President's Homes Commission, 1908), pp. 60–61.

[32] Berry, *op. cit.*, pp. 15, 19.

[33] Malcolm M. Willey and Stuart A. Rice, "The Agencies of Communication," *Recent Social Trends* (1933), pp. 172–173.

[34] "The Automobile and the Death Rate," *How to Live. A Monthly Journal of Health and Hygiene* 12:1–2 (1929); Robbins B. Stoeckel, "The Problem of Prevention of Accidents caused by the Use of Motor Vehicles," in Johns Hopkins University, School of Hygiene and Public Health, *De Lamar Lectures 1925–1926* (Baltimore, Williams and Wilkins, 1927), pp. 185–202.

[35] Stoeckel, *op. cit.*, p. 188.

[36] George Rosen, *A History of Public Health* (New York, MD Publications, 1958), pp. 237–238; *ibid.*, "Tenements and Typhus in New York City (1840–1875)," *Amer. J. Pub. Health* 62:590–593 (1972); Robert W. De Forest and Lawrence Veiller (eds.), *The Tenement House Problem*, 2 vols. (New York, Macmillan, 1903), vol. 1, pp. 71–118.

[37] John H. Pryor, "The Tenement and Tuberculosis: Apropos of the Movement for Better Housing Conditions in New York," *Charities Review* 10:440–446 (1900–1901) (see p. 443).

[38] Henry L. Shively, "Sanitary Tenements for Tuberculous Families," *The Survey* 23:885–890 (1910); Issac W. Brewer, "City Life in Relation to Tuberculosis. A Plea for Better Surroundings for Factories and Better Homes for the Working Classes," *Amer. J. Pub. Health* 3:903–914 (1913); Henry W. Farnam, *The Economic Utilization of History and Other Economic Studies* (New Haven, Yale University Press, 1913), pp. 188–189.

[39] J.B. Russell, *On the Prevention of Tuberculosis* (Boston, Wright and Potter, 1896); *A Handbook on the Prevention of Tuberculosis* (New York, Charity Organization Society, 1903).

[40] U.S. Bureau of the Census, *Historical Statistics of the United States, Colonial Times to 1957* (Washington, D.C., Government Printing Office, 1960).

[41] Emmett J. Scott, *Negro Migration During the War* (New York, Carnegie Endowment for International Peace, 1920), p. 5; *ibid.* (ed.), "Letters of Negro Migrants, 1917–18," *Journal of Negro History* 2:305–336 (1919); Sadie T. Mossell, "The Standard of Living Among One Hundred Negro Migrant Families in Philadelphia," *Annals of the American Academy of Political and Social Science* 98:169–218 (1921); August Meier and Elliott M. Rudwick, *From Plantation to Ghetto. An Interpretive History of American Negroes* (New York, Hill and Wang, 1968), p. 190.

[42] Kate H. Claghorn, "The Foreign Immigrant in New York City," *United States Industrial Commission: Reports on Immigration* (Washington, D.C., 1901), vol. 15, pp. 449 ff (Chapter IX); *Hull House Maps and Papers. A Presentation of Nationalities and Wages in a Congested District of Chicago, together with Comments and Essays on Problems Growing out of the Social Conditions by Residents of Hull House* (New York and Boston, Thomas Y. Crowell, 1895), p. 228; Jane Addams, *Twenty Years at Hull House* (New York, Macmillan, 1910), pp. 342–358; Lillian D. Wald, *The House on Henry Street* (New York, Henry Holt & Co., 1915), pp. 66, 184, 290, 310; Frank J. Bruno, *Trends in Social Work... 1874–1946* (New York, Columbia University Press, 1948).

[43] Edward T. Devine, *Misery and Its Causes* (New York, Macmillan Company, 1910), p. 55. See the section on ill health in this volume, pp. 53–112.

[44] Walter Lippmann, *Drift and Mastery. An Attempt to Diagnose the Current Unrest* (New York, Mitchell Kennerley, 1914), p. 267.

[45] Edward T. Devine, *When Social Work Was Young* (New York, Macmillan Company, 1939), p. 5.

[46] Herbert Croly, *The Promise of American Life* (New York, Macmillan Company, 1909), p. 154.

[47] Scott Nearing, *Social Adjustment* (New York, Macmillan Company, 1911).

[48] Mary Kingsbury Simkhovitch, *The City Worker's World in America* (New York, Macmillan Company, 1917), pp. 169, 176. Also see National Conference of Social Work, *Proceedings (46th Annual Session), Atlantic City, June 1–8, 1919,* Chicago, Ill. (1919), pp. III, 153–251.

[49] Charles R. Van Hise, *The Conservation of Natural Resources in the United States* (New York, Macmillan, 1910); Arthur A. Ekirch, Jr., *Man and Nature in America* (New York, Columbia University Press, 1963), pp. 81–100; William H. Harbaugh, *Power and Responsibility. The Life and Times of Theodore Roosevelt* (New York, Farrar, Straus and Cudaby, 1961), pp. 318–336.

[50] J. Pease Norton, "The Economic Advisability of Inaugurating a National Organization of Health," *J.A.M.A.,* (September 19, 1906).

[51] Among the members of the committee were Hermann Biggs, John Shaw Billings, William H. Welch, Livingston Farrand, L. Emmett Holt, A.C. Abbott, S. Adolphus Knopf, George M. Kober, Edward L. Trudeau, Henry P. Walcott, Jane Addams, Edward T. Devine, C. Loring Brace, Franklin H. Giddings, Booker T. Washington and Thomas A. Edison, in short, leaders in the fields of medicine, public health and social welfare.

[52] George Rosen, "The Committee of One Hundred on National Health and the Cam-

paign for a National Health Department, 1906–1912," *Amer. J. Pub. Health* 62:261–263 (1972).

[53] Irving Fisher, *A Report on National Vitality. Its Wastes and Conservation* (Bulletin 30 of the Committee of One Hundred on National Health) (Washington, Govt. Printing Office, 1909), pp. 126–128; *idem*: "Public Responsibility for the Health of Infants and Children," *Proceedings of the Child Conference for Research and Welfare, Held at Clark University. . . . July 6–10, 1909* (New York, G.E. Stechert & Co., 1910), vol. I, pp. 83–90.

[54] Albert G. Love and Charles B. Davenport, *Defects Found in Drafted Men* (Washington, Govt. Printing Office, 1920).

[55] Quoted on the back of Publication No. 10 of the American Association for Labor Legislation, *First National Conference on Industrial Diseases* (New York, 1910).

[56] Norton, *op. cit.*, p. 1.

[57] C.-E.A. Winslow, *The Life of Hermann M. Biggs* (Philadelphia, Lea and Febiger, 1929), p. 202.

[58] Henry B. Baker, "The Restriction and Prevention of Dangerous Diseases," *Annals of Hygiene* 5:447–460 (1890).

[59] William Warren Potter, "The Prevention of Disease: A Problem for all Physicians," *New York Medical Journal* 59:450–455 (1894) (pp. 450–451).

[60] *Ibid., op. cit.*, p. 455.

[61] Eugene H. Porter, *The Fight Against Preventable Diseases* (Albany, N.Y., New York State Department of Health, Division of Publicity and Education, (n.d.) probably 1910–1911), p. 1.

[62] Milton J. Rosenau, *Preventive Medicine and Hygiene* (New York, D. Appleton & Co., 1914), p. VII.

[63] Woods Hutchinson, *Preventable Diseases* (Boston and New York, Houghton Mifflin, 1909), chaps. XII, XIV, XVI–XIX.

[64] James Crichton-Browne, *The Prevention of Senility and A Sanitary Outlook* (London, Macmillan and Co., 1905), pp. 3–4.

[65] Newman, *op. cit.*, pp. 76–99.

[66] A detailed account of the development of microbiology and immunology, and their application for disease prevention is presented in George Rosen, *A History of Public Health* (New York, MD Publications, 1958), pp. 304–343. For the development of vaccines and sera see H.J. Parish, *A History of Immunization* (Edinburgh and London, Livingstone, 1965).

[67] Charles V. Chapin, *The Sources and Modes of Infection* (New York, John Wiley & Sons, 1910), pp. III–V.

[68] H.W. Hill, "Chairman's Address," *Public Health Papers and Reports* (APHA) 32 (Part II): 1–8 (1908); M.P. Ravenel, "The American Public Health Association. Past, Present, Future," in *A Half Century of Public Health*, ed. M.P. Ravenel (New York, American Public Health Association, 1921), pp. 13–55.

[69] The Sociological Section no longer exists. For its history see George Rosen, "The Sociological Section of the American Public Health Association, 1910–1922," *A.J.P.H.* 61:2515–2517 (1971).

[70]Walter L. Bierring, "Preventive Medicine–Its Changing Concepts, 1859–1959," *J.A.M.A.* 171:2190–2194 (1959).

[71]Since 1968 it has been the National Tuberculosis and Respiratory Disease Association.

[72]F.C.S. Bradbury, *Causal Factors in Tuberculosis* (London, National Association for the Prevention of Tuberculosis, 1933).

[73]E.G. Price, *Pennsylvania Pioneers Against Tuberculosis* (New York, National Tuberculosis Association, 1952); S.A. Knopf, *A History of the National Tuberculosis Association: The Antituberculosis Movement in the United States* (New York, National Tuberculosis Association, 1922); C.-E.A. Winslow, *The Life of Hermann M. Biggs* (Philadelphia, Lea & Febiger, 1929); R.H. Shryock, *National Tuberculosis Association, 1904–1954. A Study of the Voluntary Health Movement in the United States* (New York, National Tuberculosis Association, 1957).

[74]R. Koch, "Weitere Mittheilungen über ein Heilmittel gegen Tuberculose," *Deutsche med. Wochenschrift* 16:1029 (1890); *ibid.*: "Fortsetzung der Mittheilungen über ein Heilmittel gegen Tuberculose," *Deutsche med. Wochenschrift* 17:101 (1891). See other reports on clinical trials in this volume. For tuberculin see L. Hamman and E. Wolman, *Tuberculin in Diagnosis and Treatment* (New York, D. Appleton & Co., 1912).

[75]Georg Cornet, "Die Verbreitung der Tuberkelbacillen ausserhalb des Körpers," *Ztschr. f. Hyg. u. Infectionskr.* 5:191 (1888); C. Flügge, "Ueber Luftinfection," *Ztschr. f. Hyg. u. Infectionskr.* 30:107 (1899); Allen Krause," Essays on tuberculosis. VII. Infection by inhalation: Flügge's theory of droplet infection," *J. Outdoor Life* 15:225 (1918).

[76]George Rosen, "Historical Evolution of Primary Prevention," *Bull. N.Y. Acad. Med.* 51:9–26 (1975).

[77]Paul Ehrlich, "Aus dem Verein für innere Medicin zu Berlin. Sitzung vom 1. Mai 1882," *Deutsche med. Wochenschrift* 8:269 (1882); F. Ziehl, "Zur Färbung des Tuberkelbacillus," *Deutsche med. Wochenschr.* 8:451 (1882); B. Fränkel, "Ueber die Färbung des Koch'schen Bacillus und seine semiotische Bedeutung für die Krankheiten der Respirationsorgane," *Berl. klin. Wchnschr.* 21:193 (1884). See also H.G. Wells, L.M. DeWitt and E.R. Long, *The Chemistry of Tuberculosis* (Baltimore, Williams and Wilkins, 1923); and H.S. Willis and M.M. Cummings, *Diagnostic and Experimental Methods in Tuberculosis* (Springfield, Ill., Charles C. Thomas, 1952).

[78]C. von Pirquet, "Tuberculindiagnose durch cutane Impfung," *Berl. klin. Wchnschr.* 44:644 (1907); *ibid.*: "Der diagnostische Wert der kutanen Tuberculinreaktion bei der Tuberculose des Kindesalters auf Grund von 100 Sektionen," *Wien. klin. Wchnschr.* 20:1123 (1907); G. Mantoux, "Intradermoréaction de la tuberculine," *Compt. rend. Acad. Sci.* 147:355 (1908).

[79]Shryock, *op. cit.*, pp. 110, 168.

[80]Ida M. Cannon, *On the Social Frontier of Medicine. Pioneering in Medical Social Work* (Cambridge, Mass., Harvard University Press, 1952), p. 165.

[81]Allen K. Krause, "Tuberculosis and Public Health," *Amer. Rev. Tuberculosis* 18:271–322 (1928).

[82]O. Bollinger, "Ueber Tuberkelbacillen im Euter einer tuberculösen Kuh und über die Virulenz des Secretes einer derartig erkrankten Milchdrüse," *Ärztliches Intelligenzblatt* 30:163 (1883); Theobald Smith, "Two varieties of tubercle bacillus from mammals," *Trans. Assn. Amer. Physicians* 11:75 (1896); *ibid.*, "A comparative study of

bovine tubercle bacilli and of human bacilli from sputum," *J. Exper. Med.* 3:451–511 (1898); M.P. Ravenel, "The Intercommunicability of Human and Bovine Tuberculosis," *Univ. of Pennsylvania M. Bull.* 15:66–87 (1902); *ibid.*, "Bovine Tuberculosis as a Factor in the Causation of Human Tuberculosis," *Maryland M.J.* 47:63–72 (1904); W.H. Park and C. Krumwiede, Jr., "The relative importance of the bovine and human type of tubercle bacilli in the different forms of tuberculosis," *J.M. Research* 27:109 (1912).

[83]T.N. Bonner, *Medicine in Chicago, 1850–1950. A Chapter in the Social and Scientific Development of a City* (Madison, Wisconsin, American History Research Center, 1957), p. 48.

[84]M.J. Rosenau, *The Milk Question* (Boston and New York, Houghton Mifflin, 1912), pp. 194, 197.

[85]Philip D. Jordan, *The People's Health. A History of Public Health in Minnesota* (Saint Paul, Minnesota, Historical Society, 1953), p. 173.

[86]Robert F. Steadman, *Public Health Organization in the Chicago Region* (Chicago, Ill., University of Chicago Press, 1930), pp. 165-168, 171-176; United States Public Health Service, *The Chicago-Cook County Health Survey* (New York, Columbia University Press, 1949), p. 244.

[87]Anthony M. Lowell, Lydia B. Edwards and Carroll E. Palmer, *Tuberculosis* (Cambridge, Mass., Harvard University Press, 1969), pp. 20-21.

[88]Rosenau, *op.cit.*, p. 90.

Milk

Milk-borne Epidemics in Greater Boston

1907 Diphtheria	72 cases
1907 Scarlet fever	717 cases
1908 Typhoid fever	400 cases
1910 Scarlet fever	842 cases
1911 "Tonsillites"	2064 cases
	4095 cases

[89]Harry Linenthal, "Sanitation of Clothing Factories and Tenement-house Workrooms," in E.A. Locke (ed.), *Tuberculosis in Massachusetts* (Boston, 1908), pp. 28-36.

[90]U.S. Public Health Service, *Municipal Health Department Practice for the Year 1923 Based Upon Surveys of the 100 Largest Cities in the United States* (Public Health Bulletin No. 164) (Washington, D.C., 1926), pp. 195-196.

[91]Lowell et al., *op. cit.*, p. 13.

[92]U.S. Public Health Service, *Municipal Health Department Practice*, p. 201.

[93]Robert S. Lynd and Helen Merrell Lynd, *Middletown in Transition. A Study in Cultural Conflicts* (New York, Harcourt, Brace & Co., 1937), pp. 372-393.

[94]Margaret W. Barnard, "The X-Ray in Tuberculosis Case Finding. Preliminary Report of X-Ray Surveys of 20,000 Individuals on Home Relief in Two Districts of New York City, 1933," *Milbank Memorial Fund Quarterly* 11:1-7 (1933); H.R. Ewards, "Tuberculosis Case Finding: Studies in Mass Surveys," *Amer. Rev. Tuberculosis* 41:Suppl. 1-159 (1940); H.R. Edwards, E. Rocks and A.V. Biorklund, "The Economics of Mass Examination for Tuberculosis," *Milbank Memorial Fund Quarterly* 19:402-410 (1941); H.R. Edwards, "The Cost of Tuberculosis Control in the Department of Health, New York City, 1940," *Milbank Memorial Fund Quarterly* 21:64-79 (1943); H.E. Hilleboe and R.H. Morgan, *Mass Radiography of the Chest* (Chicago, Ill., Year Book Publishers,

1945); A.L. Blakeslee, *And the Spark Became a Flame: The Beginnings of Mass Chest X-Rays* (New York, National Tuberculosis Association, 1954).

[95] A.J. Lanza and R.J. Vane, "The Prevalence of Silicosis in the General Population and Its Effects on the Incidence of Tuberculosis," *Amer. Rev. Tuberc.* 29:8-16 (1934); L.U. Gardner, *Tuberculosis in Industry* (New York, National Tuberculosis Association, 1942); *Community Wide Chest X-ray Survey,* Public Health Service Publication No. 222 (Washington, D.C., 1952).

[96] Krause, *op. cit.,* p. 11.

[97] Lilian Brandt, "The Social Aspects of Tuberculosis Based on a Study of Statistics," *A Handbook on the Prevention of Tuberculosis* (New York, Committee on the Prevention of Tuberculosis, Charity Organization Society of the City of New York, 1903), pp. 36-38.

[98] A.K. Krause, "The Decline of Tuberculosis Mortality in the United States and the Influence of the Influenza Epidemic of 1918," *Amer. Rev. Tuberc.* 13:385-391 (1926).

[99] The phrase "in slow motion" has been borrowed from Dwight O'Hara, *Air-Borne Infection, Some Observations on its Decline* (New York, Commonwealth Fund, 1943), pp. 76-77.

[100] Wade H. Frost, "Risk of Persons in Familial Contact with Pulmonary Tuberculosis," *A.J.P.H.* 23:426-432 (1933); *Papers of Wade Hampton Frost,* Kenneth F. Maxcy, ed. (New York, Commonwealth Fund, 1941), p. 583.

[101] Ministry of Health, *On the State of the Public Health During Six Years of War* (London, H.M.S.O., 1946), pp. 59-60.

[102] W. and E. Woytinsky, "Die öffentliche Gesundheitspflege in Zahlen," *Ergebnisse der sozialen Hygiene und Gesundheitsfürsorge* 1:328-387 (1929) (see p. 361).

[103] A.K. Krause, "Antituberculosis Measures," *Amer. Rev. Tuberc.* 2:637-653 (1918) (see p. 651).

[104] Wade H. Frost, "How Much Control of Tuberculosis?" *A.J.P.H.* 27:759-766 (1973); *Papers of Wade Hampton Frost* (see ref. 100), p. 607; see also W.H. Frost, "The age selection of mortality from tuberculosis in successive decades," *Am. J. Hyg.* 30:91-96 (1939).

[105] *Recent Social Trends in the United States. Report of the President's Research Committee on Social Trends* (New York, McGraw-Hill, 1933), pp. 469, 560, 563-564, 582; John C. Gebhart, *The Health of a Neighborhood. A Social Study of the Mulberry District* (New York, Association for Improving the Condition of the Poor, 1924), pp. 5-7.

[106] U.S. Department of Commerce, Bureau of Foreign and Domestic Commerce, *Real Property Inventory* (Washington, Government Printing Office, 1934); National Resources Committee, *Technological Trends and National Policy* (1937), p. 371.

[107] Godias J. Drolet, "Epidemiology of Tuberculosis," *Clinical Tuberculosis,* ed. Benjamin Goldberg (Philadelphia, F.A. Davis & Co., 1944), vol. 1, pp. 3-70.

[108] Anthony M. Lowell, *Socio-Economic Conditions and Tuberculosis Prevalence. New York City 1949-1951* (New York, New York Tuberculosis and Health Association, 1956), pp. 16-35; Jean Downes, *An Experiment in the Control of Tuberculosis Among Negroes* (New York, Milbank Memorial Fund, 1950).

[109] Richard O. Cummings, *The American and his Food. A History of Food Habits in the United States* (Chicago, Ill., University of Chicago Press, 1940), pp. 138-228; Downes, *op. cit.,* pp. 21-25, 56; H.E. Magee, "Application of Nutrition to Public Health—Some

Lessons of the War," *British Medical Journal,* Vol. 1, pp. 475-482 (1946).

[110]*Papers of Wade Hampton Frost,* pp. 608, 611.

[111]Johannes Holm, "BCG Vaccination," *Amer. Rev. Tuberc.* 57:106 (1948).

[112]Committee on Administrative Practice, *Appraisal Form for City Health Work* (New York, American Public Health Association, 1925; 3rd edition, 1929); *ibid., Appraisal Form for Local Health Work* (New York, American Public Health Association, 1938).

[113]The American Association for the Study and Prevention of Infant Mortality was organized in 1909, as was the National Committee for Mental Hygiene. The American Society for the Control of Cancer was created in 1913, the American Heart Association in 1922, the National Foundation for Infantile Paralysis in 1938, and the American Diabetes Association in 1940.

[114]Hugh Cabot, "Is urology entitled to be regarded as a specialty?" *Trans. Amer. Urological Assn.* 5:1-10 (1911). See also pp. 14-17.

[115]Robert N. Wilson, "The Eradication of the Social Disease in Large Cities, *Transactions of the Fifteenth International Congress on Hygiene and Demography, Washington September 23-28, 1912* (Washington, D.C., 1913), vol. IV, pp. 115-126 (see p. 115).

[116]Mary A. Clark, "Venereal-Disease Control, *Report of the Committee on Municipal Health Department Practice* (Public Health Bulletin No. 136), U.S. Public Health Service (Washington, D.C., 1923).

[117]K.S.F. Credé, *Die Verhütung der Augenentzündung der Neugeborenen,* (Berlin, 1884). Today a 1-percent solution is used.

[118]Edith C. Kerby, "Causes of Blindness in Children of School Age," *Sight-Saving Review* 28:10-21 (1958); P.C. Barsam, "Specific prophylaxis of gonorrheal ophthalmia neonatorum," *New Engl. J. of Med.* 274:731 (1966); J.W. Kerr, *Ophthalmia Neonatorum: An Analysis of the Laws and Regulations Relating Thereto in Force in the United States* (Public Health Service Bulletin No. 49) (Washington, D.C., 1911).

[119]U.S. Dept. of H.E.W., Public Health Service, Center for Disease Control, *Morbidity and Mortality Annual Summary* 19, No. 53 (1970). This phenomenon has not been limited to the United States; see W.H.O., *Statistics Report* 22, No. 5 (1969); W.J. Brown et al., *Syphilis and Other Venereal Diseases* (Cambridge, Mass., Harvard University Press, 1970), pp. 38, 166-167.

[120]A.C. Curtis, "National Survey of Venereal Disease Treatment," *J.A.M.A.* 186:46-49 (1963).

[121]G.W. Mellin and M.P. Kent, "Ophthalmia neonatorum. Is prophylaxis necessary?" *Pediatrics* 22:1006-1015 (1958); J.A. Smith, "Ophthalmia neonatorum in Glasgow," *Scot. Med. J.* 14:272-276 (1969).

[122]J.R. Waters and T.M. Roulston, "Gonococcal infections in a prenatal clinic," *Amer. J. Obs. Gyn.* 103:532-536 (1969); G.W. Kraus and S.S.C. Yen, "Gonorrhea during pregnancy," *Obst. & Gyn.* 31:258-260 (1968); P.N. Sarrel and K.A. Pruett, "Symptomatic Gonorrhea during pregnancy," *Obs. & Gyn.* 32:670-673 (1968). V.G. Cave, R.D. Gloomfield et al., "Gonorrhea in the obstetric and gynecologic clinic," *J.A.M.A.* 210:309-311 (1969); A.C. Curtis, "National survey of venereal disease treatment," *J.A.M.A.* 186:46-49 (1963).

[123]L. Lehrfeld, "Limitations of Use of Silver Nitrate in Prevention of Ophthalmia Neonatorum," *J.A.M.A.* 104:1468-1469 (1935); *ibid.:* "Prophylaxis against ophthalmia neonatorum," *J.A.M.A.* 135:306 (1947).

[124] Robert J. Snowe and Catherine M. Wilfert, "Epidemic Reappearance of Gonococcal Ophthalmia Neonatorum," *Pediatrics* 51:110-114 (1973); Edward B. Shaw, "Gonorrheal ophthalmia neonatorum," *Pediatrics* 52:281-282 (1973).

[125] Fritz Schaudinn and Erich Hoffmann, "Vorläufiger Bericht über das Vorkommen von Spirochaeten in syphilitischen Krankheitsprodukten bei Papillomen," *Arbeiten aus dem kaiserlichen Gesundheitsamte, Berlin* 22:527 (1905); *ibid.:* "Ueber Spirochaeten-befunde im Lymphdrüsensaft Syphilitischer," *Deutsche med. Wchnschr.* 31:711-714 (1905); A Wassermann, A Neisser and C. Bruck, "Eine serodiagnostische Reaction bei Syphilis," *Deutsche med. Wchnschr.* 32:745-746 (1906); Paul Ehrlich and S. Hata, *Die experimentelle Chemotherapie der Spirillosen* (Berlin, Julius Springer, 1910).

[126] E. Philipp, "Die Bekämpfung der Lues bei Mutter und Kind," *Ergebnisse der Sozialen Hygiene und Gesundheitsfürsorge* 1:174-195 (1929).

[127] Brown et al., *Syphilis and Other Venereal Diseases*, pp. 109-110, 190-191.

[128] Richard A. Urquhart, "The Relation of Syphilis to Infant Mortality," *Bull. Amer. Acad. Med.* 11:161-172 (1910).

[129] For example see Erwin Meyer, "Klinische und experimentelle Untersuchungen über die Wirkung des Salvarsans auf die kongenitale Syphilis des Fötus bei Behandlung der Mutter," *Zeitschrift für Geburtshülfe und Gynäkologie* 77:20-48 (1915).

[130] Urquhart, *op. cit.*, p. 170.

[131] J. Whitridge Williams, "The Significance of Syphilis in Prenatal Care and in the Causation of Foetal Death," *Bull. Johns Hopkins Hosp.* 31:141-145 (1920) (see p. 142).

[132] J. Whitridge Williams, "The Influence of the Treatment of Syphilitic Pregnant Women Upon the Incidence of Congenital Syphilis," *Bull. Johns Hopkins Hosp.* 33:383-386 (1922); Veeder, *op. cit.* p. 146; Powers, *op. cit.*, p. 12..

[133] S.W. Trythall, "The Premarital Law: History and Survey in Michigan," *J.A.M.A.* 187:900-903 (1964).

[134] Brown et al., *Syphilis and Other Venereal Diseases*, pp. 26-27, 37, 43.

[135] C.-E.A. Winslow, "The Parent, the Strategic Point of the Present," *Bull. Amer. Acad. Med.* 11:609-611 (1910).

[136] Williams, *op. cit.* (ref. 131), p. 142; for Williams' original views see "The Limitations and Possibilities of Prenatal Care," *J.A.M.A.* 64:95-101 (1915).

[137] *Report of the Committee on Municipal Health Department Practice of the American Public Health Association*... (Public Health Bulletin, No. 136) (Washington, D.C., 1923), pp. 114-130; *Municipal Health Department Practice for the Year 1923*... (Public Health Bulletin, No. 164) (Washington, D.C., 1926), pp. 245-246; Steadman, *op. cit.*, pp. 147-148; *America's Health*. A Report to the Nation by the National Health Assembly (New York, Harper & Brothers, 1949), pp. 113-114.

[138] T. Smith, "Active Immunity Produced by So-called Balanced or Neutral Mixtures of Diphtheria Toxin and Antitoxin," *J. Experimental Medicine* 11:241-256 (1909).

[139] E. von Behring, "Ueber ein neues Diphtherieschutzmittel," *Deutsche med. Wchnschr.* 39:873-876 (1913).

[140] B. Schick, "Die Diphtherie-Hautreaktion des Menschen als Vorprobe der prophylaktischen Diphtherieheilseruminjektion," *Münchner med. Wchnschr.* 60:2608-2610 (1913).

[141] A. Zingher, "Diphtheria preventive work in the public schools of New York City," *Arch. Pediatrics* 38:336-359 (1921); W.H. Park, M.C. Schroeder and A. Zingher, "The Control of Diphtheria," *A.J.P.H.* 13:23-32 (1923).

[142] L. Baumgartner, "Relationship of age to immunological reactions," *Yale J. Biol. & Med.* 6:403-434 (1934); J. Greengard and H. Bernstein, "Passive immunity in infants and their response to diphtheria toxoid," *J.A.M.A.* 105:341-342 (1935); J.V. Cooke, "Antibody formation in early infancy against diphtheria and tetanus toxoids," *J. Pediatrics* 33:141-146 (1948); J.A. Bell, "Diphtheria immunization," *J.A.M.A.* 137:1009-1016 (1948).

[143] O. Rosenbach, *Physician versus Bacteriologist* (New York and London, Funk and Wagnalls, 1904), pp. 413-448.

[144] W.T. Russell, *The Epidemiology of Diphtheria During the Last Forty Years,* Medical Research Council, Special Report Series, No. 247 (London, H.M.S.O., 1943), pp. 27-34; Dwight O'Hara, *Air Borne Infection. Some Observations on its Decline* (New York, Commonwealth Fund, 1943), pp. 23-24; M. Burnet, *Natural History of Infectious Disease* (Cambridge, University Press, 1953), pp. 269-271.

[145] H.A. Moore and G.I. Larsen, "Present distribution of diphtheria in the United States," *Public Health Rep.* 72:537-542 (1957); T.C. Doege, C.W. Heath, and I.L. Sherman, "Diphtheria in the United States, 1959-1960," *Pediatrics* 30:194-205 (1962).

[146] Louise F. Bache, *Health Education in an American City. An Account of a Five-Year Program in Syracuse, New York* (New York, Doubleday, Doran & Co., 1934), pp. 79-80.

[147] Veeder, *op. cit.,* p. 134.

[148] F.E. Sondern, C.G. Heyd and E.H.L. Corwin (eds.), *Outline of Preventive Medicine For Medical Practitioners and Students* (New York, Paul B. Hoeber, Inc., 1929), p. XI.

[149] Harry H. Moore, "Health and Medical Practice," *Recent Social Trends in the United States. Report of the President's Research Committee on Social Trends* (New York, McGraw-Hill Book Co., 1933), pp. 1061-1113 (see pp. 1103-1104).

[150] M. Clark, *Health in the Mexican-American Culture* (Berkeley, University of California Press, 1959); Earl Koos, *The Health of Regionville. What the People Thought and Did about It* (New York, Columbia University Press, 1954); Lyle Saunders *Cultural Differences and Medical Care* (New York, Russell Sage Foundation, 1954); Margaret Mead (ed.), *Cultural Patterns and Technical Change* (New York, World Federation for Mental Health UNESCO, 1953); Benjamin Paul (ed.), *Health, Culture and Community (New York, Russell Sage Foundation, 1955);* Alexander and Dorothea Leighton, *The Navaho Door* (Cambridge, Mass., Harvard University Press, 1945); E.A. Suchman, "Sociomedical Variations Among Ethnic Groups," *Amer. J. Sociol.* 70:319-331 (1964); E.A. Suchman, "Social Patterns of Illness and Medical Care," *Journal of Health and Human Behavior* 6:2-16 (1965).

[151] National Resources Committee, *Technological Trends and National Policy including the Social Implications of New Inventions* (Washington, Government Printing Office, 1937), p. 382.

[152] Charles A. Beard (ed.), *Whither Mankind* (New York, 1928), pp. 187-207 (see p. 189).

[153] John Higham, *Strangers in the Land. Patterns of American Nativism 1860-1925* (New York, Atheneum, 1963), pp. 234-263.

[154] Kirk H. Porter (ed.), *National Party Platforms* (New York, 1924), pp. 347-348.

[155] George Rosen, *From Medical Police to Social Medicine. Essays on the History of Health Care* (New York, Science History Publications, 1974), pp. 304-327.

[156] Wilbur C. Phillips, "The Achievements and Future Possibilities of the New York Milk Committee," *Proceedings of the Child Conference for Research and Welfare, 1909, Clark University, Worcester, Mass., July 6-10, 1909* (New York, G.E. Stechert & Co., 1910), pp. 189-192.

[157] W. McDermott, K. Deuschle and C. Barnett, "Health Care Experiment at Many Farms," *Science* 175:23-31 (1972).

[158] For the history of pellagra see two good recent studies: Elizabeth W. Etheridge, *The Butterfly Caste. A Social History of Pellagra in the South* (Westport, Conn., Greenwood Publishing Co., 1972); Daphne A. Roe, *A Plague of Corn. The Social History of Pellagra* (Ithaca, N.Y., Cornell University Press, 1973).

[159] For Goldberger's work see Milton Terris (ed.): *Goldberger on Pellagra* (Baton Rouge, Louisiana State University Press, 1964).

[160] Joseph Goldberger, G.A. Wheeler, Edgar Sydenstricker, Wilford I. King et al., *A Study of Endemic Pellagra in Some Cotton-Mill Villages of South Carolina* (Hygienic Laboratory Bull. No. 153) (Washington, D.C., 1929).

[161] Rupert B. Vance, *Human Factors in Cotton Culture. A Study in the Social Geography of the American South* (Chapel Hill, University of North Carolina Press, 1929), p. 117.

[162] J.N.P. Davies, "The Decline of Pellagra in the Southern United States," *Lancet* 1:195-196 (1964).

[163] W. Dykeman and J. Stokeley, *Seeds of Southern Change. The Life of Will Alexander* (Chicago, University of Chicago Press, 1962), pp. 235-237.

[164] V.P. Sydenstricker, "The History of Pellagra, Its Recognition as a Disorder of Nutrition and Its Conquest," *American Journal of Clinical Nutrition* 6:409-416 (1958). An interesting example of synergistic prevention arising from the enrichment of bread was described by Figueroa in a study of skid-row alcoholics in Chicago. Extremely few were found to be ill with pellagra, apparently because they had been consuming fortified cereal products such as bread, doughnuts, spaghetti or sandwiches. This was in marked contrast to the prevalence of pellagra among such groups before the war. See W.G. Figueroa et al. "Lack of Avitaminosis among Alcoholics," *American Journal of Clinical Nutrition* 1:179-199 (1953).

[165] Thomas D. Clark and Albert D. Kirwan, *The South Since Appomatox. A Century of Regional Change* (New York, Oxford University Press, 1967). See particularly chaps. XV and XVIII.

[166] Roger I. Lee and Lewis W. Jones, *The Fundamentals of Good Medical Care* (Chicago, Ill., University of Chicago Press, 1933), pp. 31-46.

[167] George Rosen, "Some Substantive Limiting Conditions in Communication Between Health Officers and Medical Practitioners," *A.J.P.H.* 51:1805-1816 (1961).

[168] *Local Health Units For The Nation*, A Report by Haven Emerson with the collaboration of Martha Luginbuhl (New York, Commonwealth Fund, 1945); C.-E.A. Winslow and Ira V. Hiscock, *Community Health*, Part III. *The Practitioners Library of Medicine and Surgery*, vol. XII. *Preventive Medicine and Hygiene*, Ira V. Hiscock (ed.) (New York, D. Appleton-Century Co., 1937), pp. 305-515.

[169]Hermann Biggs, "Sanitary Science, the Medical Profession and the Public," *Medical News* 72:44-50 (1898); N.E. Ditman, "Education and its Economic Value in the Field of Preventive Medicine. The Need for a School of Sanitary Science and Public Health," *Columbia University Quarterly* Vol. X (June 1908), Supplement to No. 3, pp. 57-61; Irving Fisher, *Report on National Vitality*, pp. 55-56, 128; A.M.A. Council on Medical Education, *Report of the Sub-Committee on Hygiene, Jurisprudence and Medical Economics* Report of the Committee of One Hundred on a Standard Curriculum for Medical Colleges (Chicago, 1913).

[170]Charles V. Chapin, "Pleasures and Hopes of the Health Officer," *J.A.M.A.* 52:686-687 (1909); *idem.*, "Effective Lines of Health Work," *Providence Medical Journal* 17:12-22 (1916); *idem.*, "State Health Organization," *J.A.M.A.* 66:699-703 (1916); *idem.: A Report on State Public Health Work Based on a Survey of State Boards of Health* (Chicago, American Medical Association, 1916).

[171]Louis I. Dublin, "County Health Organization in the United States," *J.A.M.A.* 63:1739-1743 (1914).

[172]John A. Ferrell, "Careers in Public Health Service," *J.A.M.A.* 76:489-492 (1921); *ibid.*, "Measures for Increasing the Supply of Competent Health Officers," *J.A.M.A.* 77:512-416 (1921); *ibid.*, "The Trend of Preventive Medicine in the United States," *J.A.M.A.* 81:1063-1069 (1923).

[173]Rockefeller Foundation, *Annual Report* (1916), pp. 27-28.

[174]J.M. Mackintosh, *Trends of Opinion About the Public Health 1901-1951* (London, Oxford University Press, 1953), p. 5.

[175]Perrin H. Long, "The Philosophy of the Clinical Approach to Teaching in Preventive Medicine," *Proceedings of the Conference on Preventive Medicine and Health Economics,* September 30-October 4, 1946 (Ann Arbor, Michigan, School of Public Health, University of Michigan), pp. 43-51.

[176]J.A. Miller, George Baehr and E.H.L. Corwin, *Preventive Practice in Modern Medicine* (New York, Paul B. Hoeber, Inc., 1942), p. IX.

[177]Milton Terris, "Evolution of Public Health and Preventive Medicine in the United States," *A.J.P.H.* 65:161-169 (1975) (see p. 167).

[178]R.S. Lynd and H.M. Lynd, *Middletown in Transition, a Study in Cultural Conflicts* (New York, Harcourt, Brace, 1937), p. 395. See also *idem, Middletown, a Study in Contemporary American Culture* (New York, Harcourt, Brace, 1929), pp. 443-444, and 451.

[179]Carey P. McCord, *A Blind Hog's Acorns* (Chicago, Ill., Cloud, 1945), pp. 22-25.

[180]Lewellys F. Barker, "Public Health and the Future Commonwealth," *Transactions of the Conference on the Future of Public Health in the United States and the Education of Sanitarians* (Public Health Bulletin No. 126) (Washington, D.C., 1922).

[181]S. Josephine Baker, *Fighting for Life* (New York, Macmillan, 1939), p. 67.

[182]George Rosen, "The Impact of the Hospital on the Physician, the Patient and the Community," *Hospital Administration* 9:15-33 (1964); *idem: History of Public Health,* pp. 450-463.

[183]Brown et al., *Syphilis and Other Venereal Diseases,* pp. 120-128.

[184]National Resources Committee, *The Problems of a Changing Population* (Washington, Government Printing Office, 1938), pp. 7-8, 166-192; Frank W. Notestein, "The Significance of Population Trends," in *Preventive Medicine in Modern Practice,* J.A.

Miller, G. Baehr and E.H.L. Corwin (eds.) (New York, Paul B. Hoeber, 1942), pp. 28-50; George Rosen, "Health Programs for an Aging Population," in *Handbook of Social Gerontology. Societal Aspects of Aging,* Clark Tibbitts (ed.) (Chicago, Ill., University of Chicago Press, 1960), pp. 521-548 (see pp. 524-527).

[185] Hutchinson, *op. cit.,* pp. 365-366 (see ref. 63).

[186] G.L. Howe, *How To Prevent Sickness. A Handbook of Health* (New York, Harper & Brothers, 1918), pp. 141-193.

[187] Francis Carter Wood, "The Necessity of Education in the Control of Cancer," *De Lamar Lectures 1925-1926* (ref. 34), pp. 43-56.

[188] Eugene R. Kelley, "Cancer and the Health Administrator," *A.J.P.H.* 14:561-565 (1924).

[189] "The Cancer Problem from the Public Health Standpoint," *A.J.P.H.* 14:58-60(1924).

[190] Louis I. Dublin, "The Chance of Death from Cancer," *Cancer Control,* Report of the Lake Mohonk Conference (Chicago, Surgical Publishing Co., 1927), p. 274.

[191] Barbara G. Rosenkrantz, *Public Health and the State. Changing Views in Massachusetts 1842-1936* (Cambridge, Mass., Harvard University Press, 1972), pp. 161-164; George H. Bigelow and Herbert L. Lombard, *Cancer and Other Chronic Diseases in Massachusetts* (Boston, Houghton, Mifflin, 1933), pp. 100-111.

[192] Ralph C. Williams, *The United States Public Health Service 1798-1950* (Washington, D.C., Commissioned Officers Association, USPHA, 1951), p. 238; J.W. Schereschewsky, *The Course of Cancer Mortality in the Ten Original Registration States for the 21-Year Period, 1900-1920* (Public Health Bulletin, No. 155) (Washington, Government Printing Office, 1925).

[193] Harold M. Cavins, *National Health Agencies* (Washington, D.C., Public Affairs Press, 1945), p. 122.

[194] Horace Dobell, *Lectures on the Germs and Vestiges of Disease and on the Prevention of the Invasion and Fatality of Disease by Periodical Health Examination* (London, J. Churchill and Sons, 1861); George M. Gould, "A System of Personal Biologic Examinations, the Condition of Adequate Medical and Scientific Conduct of Life," *J.A.M.A.* 35:134-138 (1900); Albert Neisser, "Inwieweit können die Krankenkassen zur Bekämpfung der Geschlechtskrankheiten beitragen?" *Zeitschrift für Bekämpfung der Geschlechtskrankheiten* 2:181-247 (1904); Alexander M. Campbell, "The Necessity for a Periodical Examination of the Apparently Healthy," *Detroit Medical Journal* 4:193-195 (1904); Charles B. Slade, "Periodic Physical Examinations and Their Relation to the Practitioner," *Medical Review of Reviews* 21:338-344 (1915).

[195] E.E. Rittenhouse, "Increasing Organic Disease. The New Public Health Problem," *A.J.P.H.* 5:1130-1138 (1915).

[196] Lee K. Frankel, "Popularizing Health Conservation," Paper Read Before the American Life Convention, St. Paul, Minn., August 19, 1913; Louis I. Dublin, "The Possibility of Extending Life," An Address delivered before the Harvey Society of New York, December 16, 1922 (New York, Metropolitan Life Insurance Company, 1922); Augustus S. Knight, "Improving Human Values Through Health," Delivered at the Twenty-sixth Annual Convention of The Association of Life Insurance Presidents, New York, December 8, 1932.

[197] Haven Emerson, "The Protection of Health by Periodic Medical Examinations," *J. Mich. State Med. Soc.* 21:399 (1922). Also in his *Selected Papers* (1949), pp. 158-171.

[198] F.E. Sondern, C.G. Heyd, and E.H.L. Corwin (eds.), *Outline of Preventive Medicine* (New York, Paul B. Hoeber, 1929), pp. 1-17; Roger I. Lee and Lewis W. Jones, *The Fundamentals of Good Medical Care* (Chicago, Ill., University of Chicago Press, 1933), pp. 41-46; Miller, Baehr and Corwin, *op. cit.*, pp. 65-78 (ref. 184).

[199] Alec N. Thomson, "Periodic Health Examinations—What a County Medical Society Can Do in the Campaign," *A.J.P.H.* 14:592-594 (1924); George C. Ruhland, "What a City Health Department Can Do in a Periodic Health Examination Campaign," *A.J.P.H.* 14:594-597 (1924).

[200] Thomson, *op. cit.*, p. 592.

[201] *Medicine in the Changing Order*. Report of the New York Academy of Medicine Committee on Medicine and the Changing Order (New York, Commonwealth Fund, 1947), pp. 151-153; *Building America's Health*. A Report to the President by the President's Commission on the Health Needs of the Nation (Washington, D.C.), p. 21.

[202] Ward Darley, "What is the Next Step in Improving the Teaching of Preventive Medicine?" *News Letter*, Association of Teachers of Preventive Medicine (March, 1959).

[203] *Proceedings of the Conference on Preventive Medicine and Health Economics, September 30-October 4, 1946* (Ann Arbor, Mich., School of Public Health, University of Michigan, 1947), p. 146.

[204] For an excellent account of the early developments in the American Public Health Association see Arthur J. Viseltear, *Emergence of the Medical Care Section of the American Public Health Association, 1926-1948: A Chapter in the History of Medical Care in the United States* (Washington, D.C., American Public Health Association, 1972).

[205] "Medical Care in a National Health Program. An Official Statement of the American Public Health Association Adopted October 4, 1944," *A.J.P.H.* 34:1252-1256 (1944); "Coordination of Hospitals and Health Departments. Joint Statement of Recommendations by the American Hospital Association and the American Public Health Association," *A.J.P.H.* 38:700-708 (1948).

[206] "The Local Health Department—Services and Responsibilities," *A.J.P.H.* 41:302-307 (1951).

[207] W.S. Rankin, "Elimination of politics from public health work," *J.A.M.A.* 8:1285-1287 (1924); A.P.H.A. et al., *The First National Conference on Evaluation in Public Health* (Ann Arbor, Michigan, School of Public Health, University of Michigan, 1955).

[208] G. Rosen, "Specialization in Public Health," *A.J.P.H.* 62:624-625 (1972); Betty J. Bernstein, "Public Health—Inside or Outside the Mainstream of the Political Process? Lessons from the Passage of Medicaid," *A.J.P.H.* 60:1690-1700 (1970).

[209] N. McA. Gregg et al., "The Occurrence of Congenital Defects in Children Following Maternal Rubella During Pregnancy," *Medical Journal of Australia* 2:122-126 (1945); S. Krugman and R. Ward, "The Rubella Probelm," *Journal of Pediatrics* 44:489-498 (1954); "Rubella Vaccine Called Effective," *N.Y. Times* (March 14, 1975), p. 8.

[210] J.A. Uhr and J.B. Bauman, "Antibody Formation. I. The Suppression of Antibody Formation by Passively Administered Antibody," *J. Exp. Med.* 113:935-957 (1961); C.A. Clarke et al., "Prevention of Rh-haemolytic disease: Results of the Clinical Trial—a Combined Study from Centres in England and Baltimore," *B.M.J.* 2:907-1914 (1966); E. Borst-Eilers et al., *Prevention of Rh Sensitization, Report of a WHO Scientific Group, WHO Tech. Rep. Ser. No. 468 (Geneva, 1971).*

[211] Zena A. Stein, "Strategies for the Prevention of Mental Retardation," *Bull. N.Y.*

Acad. Med. 51:130-142 (1975).

[212]J. Lazerson, "The Prophylactic Approach to Hemophilia A," *Hosp. Pract.* 6:99-109 (1971); *ibid.,* "Home Treatment Program in Hemophilia," *Clin. Res.* 19:208 (1971).

[213]I. Moriyama, D.E. Krueger and J. Stamler, *Cardiovascular Diseases in the United States* (Cambridge, Mass., Harvard University Press, 1971), pp. 161-163.

[214]Lerner and Anderson, *Health Progress in the United States* (ref. 3), pp. 90-91; M. Silverman and P.R. Lee, *Pills, Profits and Politics* (Berkeley, University of California Press, 1974), p. 11

[215]Royal College of Physicians, London, *Smoking and Health* (New York, Pitman Publishing Co., 1962).

[216]*The Problem of Changing Food Habits. Report of the Committee on Food Habits* Bulletin, National Research Council, No. 108 (Washington, D.C., National Research Council, 1943); "Coffee Decline—Fewer Drinkers, Fewer Cups," *N.Y. Times* (March 15, 1975), p. 12.

[217]Lerner and Anderson, *op. cit.,* pp. 78-79; *National Conference on Medicine and the Federal Coal Mine Health and Safety Act of 1969. . . . .Papers and Proceedings,* Washington, D.C., June 15-18, 1970.

[218]S.P. Baker, "Injury Control," *Preventive Medicine and Public Health,* 10th ed., P.E. Sartwell, ed. (New York, Appleton-Century-Crofts, 1973), pp. 987-1005; W. Haddon, Jr., "On the Escape of Tigers: An Ecologic Note," *A.J.P.H.* 60:2229-2234 (1970); P.E. Dietz and S.P. Baker, "Evitable Injuries," *Lancet* 2:963-964 (1974).

[219]E.L. Wynder, "On the Epidemiology of Gastric Cancer: An Appraisal of the Evidence," *Racial and Geographical Factors in Tumour Incidence,* ed. A.A. Shiva (Edinburgh, Edinburgh University Press, 1967), pp. 37-66.

[220]G.N. Papanicolaou and H.F. Traut, "The diagnostic value of vaginal smears in carcinoma of the uterus," *Am. J. Obstet. Gyn.* 42:193-206 (1941).

[221]Daniel W. Cramer, "The Role of Cervical Cytology in the Declining Morbidity and Mortality of Cervical Cancer," *Cancer* 34:2018-2027 (1974).

[222]Leopold G. Koos and Alexander J. Phillips, "Summary and Recommendations of the Workshop on Uterine-Cervical Cancer," *Cancer* 33:1753-1754 (1974). This is a *Supplement* containing the Proceedings of the National Conference on Cancer Prevention and Detection, March 28-29, 1973, Bethesda, Maryland.

[223]Charles S. Cameron, "Cancer Control: Challenge or Chimera?" *Cancer* 33:402-413 (1974); also the *Proceedings* listed in the preceding reference, pp. 1703-1704.

[224]J.N. Morris, "Primary Prevention of Heart Attack," *Bull. N.Y. Acad. Med.* 51:62-74 (1975) (p. 73).

[225]W.H.O., *Expert Committee on Public Health Administration, First Report,* Technical Report Series, 55 (1952), p. 5.

[226]President's Commission on Heart Disease, Cancer and Stroke, *A National Program to Conquer Heart Disease, Cancer and Stroke* (December, 1964), vol. 1, p. 29.

[227]See for example Milbank Memorial Fund, *Report for the Year Ended December 31, 1926 with an account of the New York Health Demonstrations* (New York, Milbank Memorial Fund, 1926).

[228]"Aeromedicine: A New Specialty," *J.A.M.A.* 151:1016 (1953); T.F. Whayne, "Preventive Medicine in Medical Schools," *Archives of Environmental Health* 3:308-314

(1961); Report of the Education Committee of the American Academy of Occupational Medicine, "Board Certification in Occupational Medicine," *ibid.*, 11:272-295 (1965); John C. Hume, "Development of Residency Training in Preventive Medicine," *J.A.M.A.* 198:271 (1966).

[229] Karl Evang, *Health Service, Society and Medicine* (London, Oxford University Press, 1960), pp. 157-158.

[230] N. Piore, D. Lewis and J. Seeliger, *A Statistical Profile of Hospital Outpatient Services in the United States: Present Scope and Potential Role* (New York, Assn. for the Aid of Crippled Children, 1971), pp. 21-24.

Library of Congress Cataloging in Publication Data

Rosen, George, 1910-
  Preventive medicine in the United States, 1900-
1975.

  Includes bibliographical references.
  1. Medicine, Preventive--United States--History.
2. Public health--United States--History. I. Title. [DNLM: 1. Preventive medicine--History--U. S.
WA11 AA1 R8p]
RA445.R76   362.1'04'2   75-35978
ISBN 0-88202-103-6